1 MONTH OF FREE READING

at

www.ForgottenBooks.com

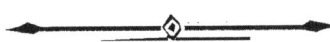

By purchasing this book you are eligible for one month membership to ForgottenBooks.com, giving you unlimited access to our entire collection of over 1,000,000 titles via our web site and mobile apps.

To claim your free month visit: www.forgottenbooks.com/free916013

* Offer is valid for 45 days from date of purchase. Terms and conditions apply.

ISBN 978-0-265-96089-9
PIBN 10916013

This book is a reproduction of an important historical work. Forgotten Books uses state-of-the-art technology to digitally reconstruct the work, preserving the original format whilst repairing imperfections present in the aged copy. In rare cases, an imperfection in the original, such as a blemish or missing page, may be replicated in our edition. We do, however, repair the vast majority of imperfections successfully; any imperfections that remain are intentionally left to preserve the state of such historical works.

Forgotten Books is a registered trademark of FB &c Ltd.
Copyright © 2018 FB &c Ltd.
FB &c Ltd, Dalton House, 60 Windsor Avenue, London, SW19 2RR.
Company number 08720141. Registered in England and Wales.

For support please visit www.forgottenbooks.com

HÆMORRHOIDS

AND

PROLAPSUS OF THE RECTUM.

HÆMORRHOIDS

AND

PROLAPSUS OF THE RECTUM:

THEIR

PATHOLOGY AND TREATMENT;

WITH ESPECIAL REFERENCE TO THE APPLICATION
OF NITRIC ACID.

WITH A CHAPTER ON THE

PAINFUL ULCER OF THE RECTUM.

BY

HENRY SMITH, F.R.C.S.,
ASSISTANT-SURGEON TO KING'S COLLEGE HOSPITAL

THIRD EDITION.

LONDON:
JOHN CHURCHILL, NEW BURLINGTON STREET.
MDCCCLXII.

PRINTED BY J. E. ADLARD, BARTHOLOMEW CLOSE.

TO

JOHN WIBLIN, Esq., M.D., F.R.C.S.,

OF SOUTHAMPTON.

My dear Wiblin,

You were pleased to express yourself to me in high terms of this work in its original form. I cannot do better than dedicate the production, in its enlarged and improved condition, to one who, during many years of friendship, has shown me great personal kindness, and who deservedly holds such an honorable position in the ranks of our Profession.

I remain,

Your faithful friend,

HENRY SMITH.

PREFACE TO THE THIRD EDITION.

In preparing a third edition of this little work, which has been so favorably received by my professional brethren, I have described and illustrated certain modes of treating Hæmorrhoids and Prolapsus which were not alluded to before, but which my more mature experience has justified me in recommending. I have, moreover, added a short, but entire chapter, on the Painful Ulcer of the Rectum, which is so often associated with, and mistaken for Hæmorrhoidal Disease.

16, Caroline Street, Bedford Square;
May, 1862.

PREFACE TO THE SECOND EDITION.

The former edition of this work consisted merely of a reprint of some papers which were originally published in the 'Medical Times and Gazette,' and which were written for the purpose of showing the value of the local application of nitric acid in certain cases of Hæmorrhoidal Disease and Prolapsus of the Rectum. In preparing this new edition, I have not confined myself mainly to an inquiry into the efficacy of one particular remedy, but have taken the opportunity to consider at some length the pathology and general treatment of the diseases in question. At the same time, the employment of nitric acid holds a prominent place in this treatise, because it is, when used with judgment and in proper cases, a very valuable agent, and one which is not sufficiently appreciated by the majority of Surgeons.

16, Caroline Street, Bedford Squáre;
February, 1860.

HÆMORRHOIDS
AND
PROLAPSUS OF THE RECTUM.

HÆMORRHOIDS.

The rectum is very liberally supplied with blood, from numerous arteries and veins ramifying over and through its structure, the greater portion of which run immediately beneath the mucous membrane, between that and the muscular tissue. Both arteries and veins freely inosculate with one another. The latter possess no valves, and empty themselves into the inferior mesenteric, which assists in forming the great vein going to circulate through the liver.

From the circumstance that the lower extremity of the rectum is so vascular, that the veins possess no valves, and that the part is being periodically subject to mechanical disturbance, it is not a matter of surprise that hæmorrhoids which in reality are composed of structure in which blood-vessels are a main element, occur so frequently as they do. It has been customary for surgical writers to divide hæmorrhoids into two distinct kinds, namely, internal and external. This is a classification from which it is as well not to depart; for, although many instances occur where it is impossible to define exactly the nature of the affection,—an internal hæmorrhoid being at one time external, from some accidental cause,—nevertheless, the pathological circumstances which exist, or which occur during the persistence of the disease, differ so widely, that it is of the utmost importance to have a right knowledge of them, in order to adopt a correct mode of treatment.

External hæmorrhoids are situated at the verge of the anus outside the sphincter, and consist of one or more tumours, composed at their first formation of dilated vessels. As the disease increases from various irritating causes, the sensitive skin around the anus becomes thickened, the cellular tissue is indurated and infiltrated, and the veins are expanded. By degrees the swelling becomes larger and harder, and does not give much annoyance when the parts are in a quiescent state; if, however, they become attacked with inflammation, the tumour increases much in size, the blood in the veins becomes coagulated, distends the coats, and not unfrequently the vessel gives way, allowing the coagulated blood to escape into the surrounding cellular tissue, where it will form a distinct sheath for itself. In the course of time the inflammatory action subsides, the blood becomes absorbed, and the tumour diminishes in size, or wholly disappears. If, however, the same irritating causes recur, and nothing effectual be adopted, the tumour again increases, the skin becomes more thickened, the cellular tissue extensively infiltrated, and in this way distinct and permanent tumours are formed around the anus, which sometimes reach a large size, consisting mainly of thickened integument and cellular tissue, enclosing veins which are at times capable of distension and repletion. In their quiet state these tumours are distinctly external; but when increased in size, they may encroach upon the cavity of the rectum, and be covered with mucous membrane, and thus be partly internal. There is not unfrequently a very œdematous condition of the cellular tissue and mucous membrane at the very verge of the anus.

With regard to the actual structure of these hæmorrhoidal tumours, it will be found, on examination, that they are composed of thickened integument, infiltrated cellular tissue, and in most cases of one or more dilated veins; if the part is at perfect rest, and has not been lately inflamed, there may be distingushed nothing beyond infiltrated tissue and thickened skin, but in cutting into an external pile, which has been somewhat irritated, or is increasing in size, there will be found either a vein considerably dilated and containing semi-coagulated blood, or the blood will have escaped from the vessel, and have become either extravasated with the surrounding cellular tissue, or have formed for itself distinct cellular sheaths. This coagulation of the blood is the reason why an incision into an external hæmorrhoidal tumour, after having become inflamed and swollen, is scarcely ever attended with bleeding; and it is one of the main pathological features in this form of tumour, and far different from what obtains in instances of the internal affection.

These external hæmorrhoids vary much in

size; sometimes the swellings not being larger than peas, at other times they are seen the size of a walnut; their presence is accompanied with unpleasant symptoms, as irritation, pain when at the closet, and a sense of bearing down, even when they are in a quiescent state; but the main source of suffering is their disposition to become suddenly enlarged and inflamed, which occurrence will arise from allowing the bowels to become constipated, from the straining attendant upon a stricture of the urethra, from excess in food and drink, or from exposure to damp and cold. Under these circumstances, the tumour, which has been hitherto small and flaccid, becomes much swollen, distended, and livid in colour. From the peculiarly sensitive character of the skin at the anus, this distension is accompanied with the most exquisite pain, and it is remarkable to witness the complete prostration with which the most powerful man is overcome when suffering from acute inflammation of external piles, and especially when the symptoms have been allowed to go on for some days, without the proper means of relief being afforded, either from obstinacy on the part of the patient, or from insufficient pathological knowledge on the part of the medical attendant.

With regard to the causes which produce this form of hæmorrhoids, there is every reason to believe that the same circumstances which tend to the production of external, induce the internal affection as well, and therefore this description will apply to both. It appears with reason that there is in some persons an hereditary disposition to hæmorrhoidal affections, and we shall every now and then see father and son, or mother and daughter, suffering one after the other in the same way. Possibly, however, this may be owing to similarity in habits, certain of which, undoubtedly, much more than others, induce these affections. Thus, those who have to sit continually at the desk, and take little walking exercise, are very liable to them; those, too, who have to stand long in certain positions, as dentists and hair-dressers, are remarkably prone to hæmorrhoids. The great source of hæmorrhoidal affections, however, is anything which prevents the healthy return of the blood from the vessels of the rectum; and thus it is that congestion of the liver, or other obstructive disease of the same viscus, is frequently associated with these affections; a constipated state of the bowels, both from the mechanical effect produced upon the vessels, and from the straining efforts necessary to unload the bowels, is found to be the cause in a vast number of cases; the pressure also caused by the pregnant womb, and by ovarian tumours, produces hæmorrhoids. In other cases, the irritation caused by the frequent taking of aperient medicines is reasonably considered to be productive of the first symptoms of the disease. Violent horse exercise, indulgence in the use of highly seasoned dishes and other indigestible food, and strong wines, together with immoderate sexual intercourse, which determines the blood more freely to the pelvic region, are each fertile sources of hæmorrhoidal affections; and it is highly necessary, before any treatment is commenced, to inquire carefully into the peculiar habits of the patient.

The treatment which should be adopted for the removal of this affection must be conducted upon the ordinary principles of surgery. In the more simple cases, little beyond a strict attention to ablution, to the regular action of the bowels, and the avoidance of those causes which are known to produce the affection, will be necessary. If the bowels are inactive, a draught of cold water before breakfast, or the use of brown bread, with a moderate amount of walking exercise, will in many instances beget a healthy tone in the intestinal canal; if, however, aperient medicines are needed, they should be of the mildest description. The compound rhubarb pill, in doses of five grains, taken occasionally before dinner, or before going to bed, is a simple and unirritating aperient. A teaspoonful of the confection of senna is also an useful and efficient aperient. If there be much irritation about the anus, an occasional dose of calomel should be taken, either before or in conjunction with these medicines. At the same time that great care is taken to provide a healthy action of the bowels, local remedies should be made use of. The ordinary lead lotion, or one made of one or two grains of sulphate of zinc to an ounce of water, should be applied to the parts morning or night; or, if a more powerful astringent application is required, the patient should use the compound gall ointment, which is an admirable agent. By these means, and by careful attention to diet, most of the ordinary cases of external piles presented to our notice may be cured, or so relieved that they will hardly excite attention.

If, however, one or more of these tumours have become enlarged and inflamed, a much more energetic treatment is required, for there is in such cases very great suffering, both local and general. If there is much swelling, and the parts are exquisitely sensitive, the patient must be confined to bed, leeches should be applied to the part, and the bleeding should be encouraged by warm fomentations; and subsequently, poultices, made either of warm bran, or of bread into which a drachm of laudanum is dropped, should be applied, and changed from time to time. Opium should be given internally, and as soon as relief from pain has been procured, the bowels should be thoroughly cleared by a saline purgative. The subsequent employment of a lotion, composed of Lotio Plumbi, Liquor Ammoniæ Acetatis, and spirits of wine, one ounce of each of the latter to six ounces of the former, will cause a shrinking and collapse of the swelling.

Not unfrequently, however, the surgeon is called to a case where most or all of these measures have been tried, and yet the patient is suffering acutely, and on examination it will be found that on one side of the anus there is a tumour of a circumscribed form, of a blue colour, and in a state of great distension. In such an instance, the suffering is produced by the accumulation and coagulation of the blood, and the proper treatment to pursue is to puncture this swelling freely with a lancet; there is an escape of coagulated or semi-fluid blood, with almost immediate relief to the painful symptoms. The subsequent application of cold water, or the lotion above mentioned, to the parts freely, will cause an almost entire removal of the disease; if, however, there is much loose and thickened skin over the site of the swelling, it should be removed with sharp scissors after the part has been punctured.

After repeated attacks of this nature, the anus becomes surrounded with distinct tumours, more or less pendulous, and liable to become swollen and inflamed; for this state of things a surgical operation is required. It is, however, a simple one, and consists of the removal of these excrescences, by sharp curved scissors. As the patient kneels upon a chair, or lies upon his side, the surgeon should lay hold of each tumour with a hooked forceps, and excise them with the scissors placed flat upon the skin.

Chloroform is rarely necessary; but if the patient is exceedingly timid, the parts may be benumbed with the ice and salt, and thus much pain may be escaped. There is generally very little bleeding, especially if great care be taken not to snip any of the mucous membrane.

Simple as this operation is, it may, in uusurgical hands, be so mismanaged, as to bring about serious results. If too much of the lax skin around the anus be taken away at the same time that the tumours are excised, the parts in healing will cicatrize so that severe contraction of the anus may follow, and the patient be placed in a most miserable plight.

The same effect is likely to be produced if the mucous membrane at the verge of the anus is interfered with to any great extent; therefore, unless there be an absolute necessity for this step, this membrane should not be cut, and only the external hæmorrhoids, with portions of the redundant integument, should be excised. Both Mr. Quain and Mr. Ashton have referred to the probability of contraction of the anus occurring after an operation improperly performed, and very recently a melancholy instance of this was presented to my notice.

A lady, in the prime of life, and suffering from external hæmorrhoids, was induced to put herself under the care of a physician-accoucheur in London, who, without hesitation, undertook to perform the necessary surgical operation upon her, in April. The cicatrization arising from the wounds made was such that, in June, complete obstruction of the bowels occurred, and her life was placed in great danger, the orifice of the anus being then nearly closed. Treatment for the stricture was then commenced, by the use of bougies, and in September she consulted me. On examination, I found the natural folds of the anus entirely destroyed, and that orifice almost obliterated by a dense, unyielding stricture, which, I ascertained by the introduction of the point of my forefinger—a step of difficulty, and painful suffering to the patient—extended for about an inch up the gut. This lady was in great dejection about herself, as she was about to return to India, and she found the introduction of bougies painful. I recommended her to have an incision made on each side of the anus, and then continue the bougies; but she had such a horror of another operation, that she would not consent to it.

It is an unpleasing task to cast blame upon a professional brother, but there cannot be a doubt that the unfortunate state of things here was the result of an ill-judged and ill-performed operation—and that, had this poor lady been under the care of a surgeon in the habit of dealing with these cases, the thing could not have occurred. It is not the first time I have witnessed most lamentable results from physicians undertaking surgical operations.

Internal hæmorrhoids are more frequent, or at all events are more often presented to the notice of the surgeon, because they are productive of much more distress, and more serious consequences are liable to result from them than from the affection situated externally; and here it will be as well to mention the symptoms which are produced by them, and which are local and general.

The first local symptom which attracts the notice of a patient suffering from internal piles, is in many cases a more or less profuse attack of hæmorrhage, which may not recur for some weeks or months, but which may persist. More or less weight and uneasiness are felt at the seat, and in course of time there will be considerable pain when the bowels are evacuated. As the swelling or swellings increase in size, the evacuation of the contents of the rectum will be more difficult and more painful; straining efforts are necessary, hence the hæmorrhoidal tumours become protruded on each visit to the closet. At the earlier periods of the disease, they may be with facility returned, but as time wears on, the pain attending defecation becomes more severe, and the process of returning the piles becomes more difficult. Not only, however, do they protrude at these times, but if the patient neglects advice, the tumours come down below the sphincter whenever he takes walking exercise; the constriction caused by the muscle produces congestion in the piles, and extreme pain, which is only relieved by their reduction, or by a spontaneous flow of blood, which, however, occurs at most inopportune periods. In addition to these symptoms, there is pain and uneasiness felt in the loins and down the thighs, more especially in females, who very often suffer most acutely, and not unfrequently have their sufferings referred to that prolific storehouse of morbid phenomena, the womb. There is, moreover, a considerable discharge of mucus or muco-purulent fluid from the anus; the bladder is rendered at times very irritable, and retention of urine not unfrequently takes place.

Patients who suffer from internal hæmorrhoids, are liable to get them inflamed from some exciting cause, such as an excess at the table, or great irritation of the bowels, and then the symptoms are extremely severe; the tumours become inflamed, gorged with blood, protrude beyond the anus, and become constricted by the sphincter. Violent pains are experienced in the pelvic region, and there is a high state of constitutional disturbance, denoted by flushed face, furred tongue, rapid and wiry pulse, and extreme restlessness. If these symptoms are not relieved, either by the accidental induction of bleeding, or by surgical assistance, the congestion and inflammation increase, and to such an extent, that mortification of the hæmorrhoidal masses ensues, and thus is produced a natural cure; but, on the other hand, it is not desirable to encourage this rude attempt at cure, for death may occur from the violent action set up. Dr. Bushe mentions having seen such a case occur.

When internal hæmorrhoids have existed for a length of time, the general health becomes much influenced, the patient complains of indigestion, flatulence, and inability to follow his ordinary occupation or amusement; moreover, if, as is frequently the case, the disease be attended with periodical bleedings, the face becomes blanched, the pulse weak and rapid, and other well-known symptoms of loss of blood ensue. This is the most serious condition connected with hæmorrhoids of long standing, and hence the reason why it is most important to adopt the proper treatment at an early period of these affections.

Internal hæmorrhoids present various appearances. On making an examination of a patient who suffers from the milder form of the affection, the veins of the lower extremity of the rectum, just within the anus, will be found enlarged and distended, forming small fusiform tumours, of a dark-blue colour, covered by a somewhat thickened mucous membrane. In other instances, and especially where the patient complains of bleeding and sense of weight, with scarcely any protrusion, the inferior extremity of the rectum, for an inch or more, will be found to be highly congested and vascular; the mucous membrane having, here and there, distinct patches or morbid vascularity, from which, through a speculum, which it is necessary to use in such cases, blood of an arterial colour will be seen to issue. This is the condition which the late Dr. Houston, of Dublin, likened to the diseased lining membrane of the palpebræ, in cases of chronic conjunctivis. In the majority of instances, however, of internal hæmorrhoids, one or more distinct tumours, of a rounded or oblong form, will be seen to fill up, as it were, the orifice of the anus. In some cases, their character and size can be ascertained by an ordinary inspection, but it is always best, in order to arrive at a proper diagnosis, to throw up the bowel an injection of warm water, and allow it to be discharged before the examination is made; by this means the tumours are brought fairly down. There are frequently two or three distinct tumours, varying from the size of a fourpenny-piece to that of a walnut. In one case the diseased part presents a bright-red appearance, easily bleeds when touched, and is sessile, and not very raised; in another case the tumour is large, prominent, of a deep-blue or reddish-brown colour, having a broad base, or being attached by a narrower peduncle, and does not bleed when touched; in these cases the vessels appear to be largely dilated, the mucous membrane covering them being shining and tense, or thick, granular, and slightly ulcerated. Besides these appearances, portions of the mucous membrane, highly vascular and thickened, may be prolapsed at one or more points, as a consequence of the mechanical weight of the internal tumours. In by far the majority of cases of long-standing piles, the integument surrounding the anus is in an unhealthy condition, being much thickened, and now and then forming a distinct ring, or long pendulous flaps.

There is one point of importance connected with the seat of internal hæmorrhoids which should not be overlooked, but which, as far as I am aware, has not been mentioned by any writer on this subject. The circumstance I refer to is this—that occasionally instances are met with where the hæmorrhoidal tumours are placed as it were in separate rows, so that two or three distinct masses exist near the anus, and about half an inch or more above. Other tumours of a similar nature are disposed just in the same way. There are one or two specimens indicating this in the Museum of the Royal College of Surgeons. This is a condition of practical importance, for it shows how necessary it is to make a most thorough examination of a person suffering from internal piles. Cases every now and then occur where the ligature has been applied to one or more internal tumours presenting themselves at the anus; and, as the operator is thinking his proceedings are satisfactorily terminated, the patient makes some violent straining effort, and another tumour or series of tumours, which have escaped notice hitherto, are forced into view. These are formed higher up in the bowel, and do not generally protrude; but if a satisfactory cure is expected, they must not be left alone.

As regards the structure of internal hæmorrhoids—when first forming, they are composed, in many instances, simply of dilated veins; in others of dilated veins and arteries too. As the diseased condition increases, the cellular tissue, in connexion with the vessels, becomes thickened and infiltrated in a more or less circumscribed space; the mucous membrane also becomes thickened, and is bulged out by the increase in the size of the vessels, and thus distinct tumours are formed. The surface of the mucous membrane becomes also exceedingly vascular. On making a section of the lower part of the rectum, in cases of old standing piles, the veins will be found to be greatly dilated, sometimes partially and irregularly, so that there will be the appearance of distinct cysts. In other instances the dilated vessels will be found to be filled with coagulated blood and fibrine. In those cases where the hæmorrhoids are of a very bright red colour and sessile, not unlike a strawberry in appearance, and easily bleeding, the structure consists mainly of a series of small arterial ramifications; but where the tumours are of a darker colour, and like a mulberry, they are composed of veins to a large extent, although, no doubt, the arteries enter as well into their formation, and to a considerable extent; for when their mucous covering is pricked or incised, the blood which flows is of an arterial hue. In those cases of very long standing, and where the tumour has become very large, and has been submitted to great irritation, a section will reveal scarcely anything beyond a mass of highly condensed and thickened cellular tissue, with some vessels penetrating the base of the tumour.

The treatment of internal hæmorrhoids requires more consideration than that which is adopted for the disease when situated externally. In the cases where the piles have not existed long, are not large, and give only temporary annoyance, much may be done by the patient paying simple attention to his habits, and avoiding those exciting causes which engender the disease. If it is ascertained that a sedentary life has produced the affection, by determining the blood to the rectum, the patient should take as much walking exercise as possible; if the bowels are sluggish, their action should be encouraged by a compound rhubarb pill, or by a teaspoonful of the confection of senna; and a quarter or half a pint of cold water, or of infusion of quassia, should be thrown up the rectum daily. Dietetic rules must be strictly attended to; for many patients, especially those who are robust, and whose circulation is sluggish, will tell us that they feel much more annoyance from piles after they have been dining out, or have taken larger quantities of wine than usual. Hence the necessity of those who suffer from internal hæmorrhoids to abstain as much as possible from the pleasures of the table. Women in an advanced state of pregnancy, suffering from the irritation of piles, should be very careful about the condition of their bowels, and should keep the horizontal posture as much as possible.

When internal hæmorrhoids increase to such an extent as to protrude at the closet, and produce considerable pain and bleeding, greater precautions and more decided treatment are needful. The bowels should never be allowed to become costive, so as to necessitate straining efforts; the protruded parts should be carefully sponged with cold water, or with a strong infusion of quássia, or of decoction of oak-bark and alum, in the proportion of half a drachm of the salt to twelve ounces of the former, and should be carefully returned by the patient; or, instead of these lotions, the gall ointment may be smeared over the piles with great benefit. The bleeding, which is often very annoying, may be checked by an injection of sulphate of iron and water in the proportion of one to two grains of the former, to an ounce of the latter; or if necessary, a lotion of tannin in the proportion of eight grains to an ounce may be used; but it must be borne in mind, that a moderate amount of bleeding in persons who live high, and whose vascular system is excited, is beneficial than otherwise, and should not be interfered with; the popular notion as to bleeding from piles being salutary, is by no means incorrect when applied to certain cases. When, however, the hæmorrhage arises from some peculiar pathological change in the tumour, such as ulceration or excessive vascularity of the mucous membrane; and when it becomes continuous, and goes on to such an extent as to interfere with the patient's health, producing a pallid face, a weak pulse, and irritable heart, it should be put a stop to.

A very common internal remedy for piles is the confection of black pepper, in the dose of a drachm twice a day. It may be given by itself; or, as I often use it, mixed with an equal part of confection of senna; it is difficult to say how the remedy acts; but it certainly does good not only in this affection, but it is highly serviceable in other affections of the rectum, and especially in those cases where the wounds become sluggish in healing after the operations for fistula, or for fissure of the anus.

From the close connexion between the neck of the bladder and the rectum, it follows that the affections of the former viscus, together with those of the prostate gland, or urethra, will influence the rectum much; and thus, in middle-aged or elderly men, special inquiry should be directed to these parts; for not unfrequently hæmorrhoids and prolapse of the rectum will be found to be much aggravated, if not caused, by the violent straining efforts made in the difficult attempts to pass water. If stricture exists, the urethra must be dilated before there can be any hope of curing the piles; and even if there be not any stricture, and yet there be a loss of the contractile power of the bladder from debility or old age, this viscus should be artificially emptied by the catheter.

When internal piles become inflamed and protruded beyond the sphincter, the patient will suffer much, both locally and constitutionally; he must be confined to bed, and the piles, if possible, should be carefully returned by the surgeon; but, if this be a work of great difficulty from swelling and congestion, leeches should be applied, and subsequently warm fomentations and poultices. Ice, locally applied in a bladder, is a valuable agent to diminish inflammation and pain; opium should also be given in full doses. Any operation which may be considered advisable should not be put in force whilst the hæmorrhoids are in a state of actual inflammation. Sometimes, as I have before stated, the constriction of the sphincter produces sloughing, and a spontaneous cure takes place; if this is occurring, the process must be expedited by the liberal use of warm bathing and poulticing, and pain must be conquered by the administration of opium.

By the adoption and right application of these remedial measures a large proportion of cases of internal hæmorrhoids may be cured, or relieved to so great a degree as to prevent annoyance; but many of those cases which are presented to the notice of the surgeon have existed so long, have reached such a size, and are productive of such troublesome and even serious symptoms, that some active surgical interference is required, in order to bring about a cure or produce efficient relief. Originally, the usual remedy in aggravated cases was the excision of the diseased part, and it was a remedy accompanied with little pain or difficulty; but the danger of hæmorrhage proved to be so great, that, after the sacrifice of several lives, the practice has almost been abandoned. It is necessary, even when the excision of external piles is being performed, to take care that the mucous membrane be not too freely clipped, otherwise dangerous bleeding may result. I saw a gentleman nearly lose his life from the inclusion of a portion of mucous membrane in the blades of the scissors during an operation for external hæmorrhoids—the operation was done at two p.m., and at six I was sent for, and found that he had been bleeding profusely.*

The removal of internal hæmorrhoids by the ligature, is the method which has been commonly followed of late years; and it is necessary to devote more consideration to this part of the subject, as this treatment is most generally adopted by the very best surgeons of the day. The manner in which the ligature acts, is by the strangulation of the vessels which supply and form the tumour; the result is sloughing of the tied part, and its subsequent removal in a few days; a sore is left on the separation of the thread, and this, in healing, cicatrizes, contracts, and braces up the neighbouring tissues, so that, in addition to the bodily removal of the tumours, the tendency to their reproduction, or to any protrusion of the mucous membrane, is diminished by the result of this process.

It is undeniable that the ligature is an admirable remedy; and that it is calculated, when properly applied, to bring about a cure in the worst forms of internal hæmorrhoids; but its

* I shall speak in a future part of this work of a plan combined of excision and the use of nitric acid.

employment is open to some objections, which it is right to mention.

In the first place, it is necessary that those who undergo the operation by the ligature, should be confined to their bed for some days; in the next place, the process of applying the ligature is attended sometimes with considerable suffering. In some conditions of the constitution, a low inflammation of an erysipelatous character may ensue and spread along the intestinal tract, producing the most severe and even serious symptoms. Pyæmia also has occasionally ensued after this operation, and has destroyed life. Sir Benjamin Brodie, Sir Astley Cooper, Mr. Henry Lee, and others, have mentioned fatal cases from this cause. Tetanus has also carried off patients who have undergone this operation.

I dwell more particularly upon these untoward events, because it is rather the fashion to look upon the operation by ligature as a perfectly safe proceeding. Mr. Syme has even gone so far, as to state his opinion that "it may be used without the slightest risk of any serious inconvenience."* Now I do not hesitate to say, that

* 'On Diseases of the Rectum,' Third Edition, p. 8.

no surgeon who is acquainted with the literature of this subject is justified in making a statement so strong as this, even though his own experience of the operation may have been of the most favorable kind.

I hope I shall not be looked upon, from the previous remarks, as an opponent of the ligature; on the contrary, I believe that this proceeding is indispensable in certain cases; that when properly applied, and followed by proper treatment, it is an admirable remedy, and generally productive of a cure; and, as regards danger to life, although there is some risk, with which the patient should be made acquainted, it is undoubtedly small; and this may be lessened by taking care not to operate on persons who are much broken down in health, or suffering from any organic disease of the intestines, liver, or kidneys.

The ligature is adapted for those cases where the hæmorrhoidal tumours are large, well defined, and prominent, and where they present a dark-blue appearance, as though they consisted mainly of venous ramifications. It is moreover proper in those instances of internal hæmorrhoids, where the tumours are perhaps of a bright-red colour and easily bleed—but their dependent portions, from continued prolapse and irritation, and from existing many years, have become very much thickened and indurated. It should also be used in those cases where there is a considerable amount of prolapsus attending upon the original affection; and if an alarming amount of hæmorrhage has been the most prominent symptom, and this bleeding proceed from a distinct tumour, the ligature should undoubtedly be applied.

This proceeding is also well adapted for those cases where patients are exceedingly sensitive and nervous, and will not allow more than one operation to be performed; in one of the last cases I applied the ligature; the disease might have been destroyed by nitric acid, but the patient was very timid, and I thought it prudent to adopt a measure which would only be required once.

The operation is performed in the following manner :—The patient, who has previously had an enema of warm water, so as thoroughly to bring down the hæmorrhoidal tumours, either kneels down upon an arm-chair, or lies on his side upon a bed or sofa. An assistant separates the buttocks, whereupon the surgeon lays hold, with a long pair of forceps, or vulsellum, of the tumour which is to be operated on. The assistant makes traction with the instrument, so as to expose and isolate the tumour as much as possible. The operator then, by means of a well curved needle, set in a strong handle, passes a double thread of strong silk or twine, through the base of the mass; and, having cut the thread and removed the needle, ties each half of the tumour as tightly as possible. The ends of the ligatures are cut off close to the knot, and the protruded parts are returned within the bowel, and the operation is finished. It is better to notch the circumference of the tumour at the point where the ligature will fall before it is tied, as the separation will take place earlier; for this hint I am indebted to Mr. Curling. If there are two or three distinct hæmorrhoidal tumours, each of them must be operated upon in the manner I have described.

If there be much loose integument about the anus, the redundancy should be removed with the scissors. Too much, of course, should not be taken away, as inconvenient contraction might take place; but the surgeon who understands his business will not be likely to fall into an error of this kind. If the loose flaps of thickened integument, which are so frequently seen in connexion with hæmorrhoids, are not taken away by the scissors, there is a probability that the cure will not be perfect. Several cases have lately been under my care, where the ligature had been applied by various surgeons, and where the disease had returned. In some of these cases, the external folds of integument had not been removed; and I cannot help believing that this neglect had been the cause of the failure of the operations.

The proceedings above detailed are finished in a few minutes. If the patient be courageous and determined, I would rather operate without giving him choloroform; but if he is highly sensitive and timid, it would be better that he should inhale it, as the pain in such instances may be very severe.

The patient must keep his bed for some days after the operation. A full dose of opium must be given the first night, so that pain may be prevented and the bowels be confined. If there be much pain about the seat of operation, ice applied in a bladder continuously will give great relief. Retention of urine is apt to follow this operation, and when present must be relieved by the catheter. It is desirable to keep the bowels quiet for three or four days, if possible, and then to obtain an evacuation by a dose of castor-oil. Very likely the ligatures will separate on the first action of the bowels; at all events, they generally come away on the fifth or sixth day. Some pain is felt in the part for a few days afterwards, and during this time the patient should keep quiet. Convalescence may be expected in a fortnight from the time of the operation.

Before leaving this part of the subject, I will give illustrations of the treatment by ligature.

CASE I.—A gentleman, aged forty-nine, was sent to me, by Mr. Giraud, of Faversham, in May last. He informed me that he had suffered from hæmorrhoids for fifteen years, but that he had only been troubled with protrusion for two years, during which period he has been much annoyed, so that he was compelled to get a spring-pad—which closed the orifice of the bowel, and gave some relief, but only partially, as on walking much protrusion occurred, although the instrument was kept on. Severe hæmorrhage had also been an occasional symptom.

On examining this gentleman, I found one distinct hæmorrhoidal tumour on the left side. It was of large size, of a blue, livid colour, much like a mulberry in appearance, and without any red vascular points, or arterial varices, the mucous membrane not being ulcerated. The tumour was quite isolated, and evidently composed mainly of venous ramifications. The integument around the anus was much thickened, and elongated in flaps. The general health was good; and there being no contra-indication, I recommended the use of the ligature.

The bowels having been previously well cleared out, and the hæmorrhoidal tumour well protruded, the ligature was applied June 1st. Just as I had completed the process, the patient, who was not under the influence of chloroform, made some violent expulsive efforts, and by this means forced down another small hæmorrhoidal tumour. I therefore put a ligature through this; I then excised with the scissors the redundant and thickened skin around the anus, and completed the operation.

No retention of urine followed this proceeding; but there was much flatulent distension for thirty-six hours, and sharp febrile symptoms, which lasted three days; there was more or less pain about the rectum until the seventh day, when the ligatures separated. After this all symptoms ceased, and he left London in another week convalescent.

In this case, although the result was very favorable, the patient suffered much more than usual; and in the greater number of cases I have met with, those who have undergone this operation have suffered but little, and have been able to move about in a week. The following two cases illustrate the usually rapid recovery after the ligature has been properly applied:

CASE II.—An officer, aged twenty-four, was sent to me by Mr. Melville Jones, of the Royal Artillery, in March, 1860. He had suffered for more than six years from protrusion and from bleeding. On examination, I found that a large internal hæmorrhoidal tumour could be protruded without much effort. It was nearly as big as a walnut, was of a florid, highly vascular character, and had a broad base, and it was a source of serious annoyance to the patient. As it would have been useless to attempt to destroy this tumour with caustic, and as there was no contra-indication to the operation, I recommended the ligature, and accordingly having taken the precaution to unload the patient's bowels well, I performed the operation on April 1st, in the usual manner; the patient did not have chloroform, felt scarcely any pain at the time and had no suffering afterwards. The bowels were kept quiet until the 5th, when they were acted upon by castor-oil; the ligature came away, there was no protrusion whatever, and the patient left for Woolwich on the 7th.

CASE III.—Dr. C—, aged fifty, consulted me in June, 1860. Had suffered from protrusion and bleeding from the rectum for fifteen years, and he had been seriously annoyed by the depressing effect of his disease. He had had nitric acid applied on one or two occasions, and one or two ligatures had also been used, but latterly the protrusion not only took place when he was at the closet, but it occurred whilst he was walking.

On examination, I found a mass of protrusion consisting of three distinct portions of mucous membrane, the smallest tumour being the size of a nut, the largest nearly that of a small egg; the mucous membrane covering this tumour was thick and non-vascular, and it was evident at a glance that the nitric acid would not suit this case; so I strongly recommended the ligature.

June 24th, I performed the operation, having tied the three tumours separately; the patient scarcely complained of any pain at the time, but afterwards he suffered for several hours, and was compelled to take two grains of opium which gave relief. He had no bad symptom, and the bowels were kept confined until the 28th, when they were acted on by castor-oil without pain or protrusion, and no trace of the disease could be seen. Next day this gentleman was so well as to be able to take a drive in his carriage.

In neither of the cases mentioned had the health of the patients been materially interfered with, and therefore a speedy recovery might have been anticipated; and in such cases, those who submit to this operation may with confidence be assured that, in all probability, they will be convalescent in a week. The suffering produced by the operation is also frequently so slight, that it is difficult to make some patients keep to their bed. .

When, however, the disease has existed in a very severe form for several years, and the general powers have been much shattered by continual hæmorrhages, the operation of the ligature, although terminating in the most gratifying results, will probably be followed by a more or less protracted convalescence, for the reason that the system, when rendered weak and irritable by loss of blood, is unable to stand up so well against any surgical proceeding; and perhaps a period of three or four weeks may elapse before the patient can be pronounced well, or is able to go out. I have met with a few such instances, but the patients were either of large frame or had been terribly shaken by bleeding. The following case is related, both for showing the efficacy of the ligature and illustrating the severe effects which may be produced by neglected hæmorrhoids :

CASE IV.—Mr. J—, aged forty-seven, consulted me, January 16th, 1861. He informed me that he had suffered from hæmorrhoids attended with severe bleeding for ten years.

He had formerly been a very stout man, of florid complexion, and used to be subject to fulness about the head, which was relieved by the periodical and free bleeding from the rectum; therefore it was not interfered with, but has been allowed to go on.

I scarcely have ever seen a patient whose aspect more strikingly indicated the effects of long continued bleeding. His face and hands were pale and waxy, the voice was weak, and his gait was feeble; the action of the heart was very weak, pulse diminished to a thread, respiration was difficult, and there was a great indisposition to any exertion. He told me that the present attack of hæmorrhage had been continuous for three weeks, and that the quantity lost had been immense.

On examination, I found that there were two large internal

hæmorrhoids with distinct pedicles, and I recommended the ligature on the following day, when I operated on the patient with the assistance of Mr. Chapman, of Richmond. Before commencing, I gave an injection, which brought the parts well down, and I then discovered a third smaller and very vascular tumour seated higher up. I placed ligatures around each of the diseased masses. On the 22nd, five days after the operation, the bowels were opened by castor oil, without any bleeding or protrusion; no bad symptoms whatever occurred, and the patient gradually recovered his health.

Although it is rare to see so bad a case as this, it is, to a certain extent, the type of many cases of neglected hæmorrhoids, attended with severe hæmorrhage. The patients, as in this instance, have been robust men, have felt relieved by the periodical bleedings, and have, under the fallacious assumption that such losses of blood are beneficial to the system, allowed them to go on to such an extent, that both the physical and mental energies have been reduced to a very serious degree. I was lately called by Dr. Beaman to see a middle-aged lady who had been suffering from these periodical hæmorrhages from the rectum, to such an extent that she could not move about without great difficulty; and an œdematous condition of the limbs had shown itself.

The only treatment to be adopted in these cases is to resort to the ligature; but it is needful to be very careful in making an examination before the operation is completed, as the bleeding may come from one particular spot, which may be readily overlooked, and the operation may fail, although one or more prominent tumours have been tied. If the patient will not submit to the ligature, nitric acid may be resorted to, and with great temporary advantage; but in these cases of severe hæmorrhage, I have generally found that the symptoms return after a time; and in two very well-marked instances which have recently been under my care, I was compelled to resort to the ligature, after having given the nitric acid the most careful trial.

Before leaving this part of my subject, I must now repeat my previous statement with regard to the utility of the ligature. Within the last few years, I have had numerous opportunities of practising this operation, and I can truly say that in no single case have I experienced any uneasiness with regard to the result. The pain attending the operation, when skilfully performed, and when the hæmorrhoidal tumours are well brought down, is generally slight; in some instances, there is scarcely any suffering after the operation, and in those cases where severe pain does follow, it may be speedily relieved. I have only met with one case where retention of urine ensued, and in no instance have I met with any abdominal tenderness. In September last I was somewhat startled, on going to see a gentleman on whom I had operated two or three days previously, and finding him very feverish and complaining of pain in the wrists and elbows; but in twenty-four hours I found, to my great relief, that it was an attack of rheumatic inflammation, instead of pyæmia. The freedom from retention of urine, and from pain after the operation, is attributable, in a great measure, to the practice invariably adopted by me, of introducing a suppository, composed of six or eight grains of Pil. Saponis co., and as many of Extract Hyoscyami into the rectum, as the last step of the process.

Before proceeding further, I may state that there are cases every now and then to be met with where internal hæmorrhoids, and especially those attended with periodical bleeding, seem to be a salutary guard against other diseases, and therefore should not be interfered with, especially by any decided measures, as the ligature. I not unfrequently see cases in the persons of robust, florid people, who live well, and take little exercise, in whom it would be highly imprudent to repress the periodical bleeding from the rectum. Other instances also are met with where some disease of the brain, lungs, or stomach had existed prior to the occurrence of the hæmorrhoids, and where it had apparently become arrested by the occasional loss of blood from the rectum. In such instances, it will be most prudent to avoid surgical interference at all; if, however, from local suffering and annoyance, some operative measure becomes necessary, that mode of proceeding by which the results are produced most gradually should be adopted, and the patient should be enjoined afterwards to pay strict attention to diet and exercise, and to keep the bowels free, so as to compensate in some way for the removal of that which has been, in all probability, a source of relief to some congested or labouring organ.

Excellent, as a means of cure, though the

ligature may be for the more severe cases of internal hæmorrhoids, it is not necessary in many instances which, nevertheless, require active surgical interference; and if we possess any means by which the disease may be cured or remedied without the confinement, and that certain amount of risk which is associated with the practice of the ligature, we are bound to consider in what cases it may be employed.

Nitric acid was strongly recommended by the late Dr. Houston, of Dublin, as a means of getting rid of some forms of internal hæmorrhoids; and it is somewhat curious that, although his paper was published in the 'Dublin Quarterly Journal' more than fifteen years since, and Mr. Fergusson, in his 'Practical Surgery,' soon afterwards drew especial attention to the subject, the use of the agent was comparatively unknown, or, at all events, has not had that attention paid to it which it deserves. I have been in the habit of using the strong nitric acid in certain cases of hæmorrhoidal affections for a period of ten years, and some of the observations and cases following were originally published in the columns of the

'Medical Times and Gazette,' in separate papers. Mr. Henry Lee has incorporated with his " Surgical and Pathological Essays" an admirable paper on this subject, and has spoken highly of the plan of treatment which I am now about to consider.

I have stated, whilst describing the nature of internal hæmorrhoidal diseases, that the condition in which they are found varies. I have endeavoured to point out those cases to which the operation of the ligature is applicable, and have stated that this practice is proper and justifiable in those instances where the tumours are large, mainly composed of tissues in which the veins predominate, and have become indurated. There are, however, other instances where the hæmorrhoidal tumours are small or moderate in size, and where they are evidently composed of morbid texture, in which the small arteries rather than the veins are interested, as shown by their bright florid aspect, and their tendency to pour out arterial blood whenever the patient is at the closet, or when the tumours are handled. These tumours are generally not very prominent. They produce exceeding annoyance, and indeed, prove more destructive to the health, as they generally yield a great deal of blood. Now, in such cases, the ligature will undoubtedly be as effective as in the other instances before described; but this proceeding is not necessary, as the local use of the nitric acid is so eminently suited to them. The relief which one single application of the acid gives in these cases is remarkable, and an excellent cure may be effected, if the whole of the diseased texture be subject to its action.

About these particular kind of cases, there is no doubt in the mind of any surgeon who has seen the nitric acid applied in a proper manner. There is however a mixed class of cases where the remedy is an uncertain one, but in which, nevertheless, the surgeon is justified in trying it, and where I sometimes have succeeded when I little expected it. I refer to those cases where there is a hæmorrhoidal mass, consisting perhaps of one tumour, mainly composed of venous ramifications, and of a bluish colour, with one or more presenting the characters of the florid sessile pile; or one portion of the tumour or tumours may present the dark blue appearance and thickened membrane, and another portion of it may be brightly vascular, have its mucous covering granular and slightly ulcerated. In this kind of mixed case, I do not hesitate to try the acid if the patient is particularly desirous, but I make a point of stating that it is impossible to depend upon any curative action in such, although in some instances the remedy has acted most efficiently.

To apply the agent to those cases where the tumours are large and indurated, and have a deep blue colour, would be perfectly useless, and only bring discredit upon the nitric acid as a means of cure in other kinds of hæmorrhoidal disease. I particularly wish to point this out, as it is very probable that some of my brethren think that I am an enthusiast with regard to the use of this remedy, and recommend it too strongly. On the contrary, I always urge upon the patient the necessity and propriety of the ligature in such, and even in the more doubtful cases just alluded to. It is not necessary, because a surgeon may have reason to adopt, with confidence, a particular kind of remedy, that he should be an enthusiast, or should be blind to the value of those other means which are generally recognised as suitable and efficient.

It is, however, in that class of cases not unfrequently met with, where there is not so much any decided hæmorrhoidal tumour, but where there is a generally congested and relaxed condition of the mucous membrane of the rectum, attended with bleeding to a greater or less extent, that the nitric acids act so beneficially. Dr. Houston has compared this condition of the rectum not inaptly to that of the thickened conjunctiva after long-continued ophthalmia. The application of the acid to the diseased points from which the bleeding proceeds will soon remedy all the bad symptoms.

Having described the cases to which this agent is applicable, it is fitting that something should be said about its mode of action.

When the strong nitric acid is applied in a very limited degree to the vascular mucous membrane, or granular tumour, I believe it acts beneficially, much in the same way as does the nitrate of silver, or other powerful caustic, when applied to a spongy, irritable sore on the leg, by altering the condition of the minute vessels, contracting them, and perhaps causing coagulation of the blood in them. When however it is used more freely, superficial destruction of the tissue to which it is applied takes place, an eschar forms, this is in time removed, cicatrization necessarily ensues, vessels which formerly bled are closed up, the tissues generally are braced up and contracted, and probably adhesion is formed between the mucous and muscular tissue of the gut. By further applications of the acid to the same part, the morbid texture may be actually destroyed; and hence the remedy, powerful as it is, requires great care in its use.

I will now describe the manner in which the acid should be applied.

The bowels having been well evacuated some hours previously, the diseased portion to which the application is going to be made should be well exposed, by making the patient sit over hot water for some few minutes; or if this is not sufficient, an enema of water should be thrown up the rectum, and the hæmorrhoidal disease will be brought well into view. The part to which the acid is to be applied, should then be carefully wiped with a portion of lint.

The surgeon then dips the extremity of a small, flat piece of wood into the nitric acid, and touches the diseased surface carefully with it. The part touched, and the neighbouring mucous membrane is well smeared with oil, and the whole of the exposed part is returned within the orifice.

There are certain details connected with the application of this agent which require attention. Thus, the acid which is used should be the strongest and purest which can be obtained. I have generally employed the colourless acid, but sometimes I have thought it desirable to use the brown *fuming* nitrous acid, which acts more energetically. I have used for the most part a piece of wood as the means of carrying the acid on to the part, but some object to it as liable to be acted upon by the agent, and therefore recommend a glass rod or brush, both of which suffice very well, but I do not think it much matters.

It is important to touch the part only lightly, especially in those cases of vascular piles where bleeding easily takes places; for the blood, escaping and mixing with the acid, will in a measure neutralize its effects. I also lay great stress upon the necessity of wiping the diseased part with lint, previous to applying the acid, for there is always a certain amount of mucus covering these tumours, and unless this be removed, the nitric acid will not act efficiently.

I have recommended that the diseased parts should be brought down, either by the action of an enema, or by the efforts of the patient sitting over warm water; but there are cases where it will be difficult and unpleasant to effect this object in either way, and in this case I adopt the plan recommended many years since by Mr. Fergusson, of using a silvered glass speculum, by the introduction of which a good view of the hæmorrhoidal tumour may be had, and the nitric acid can be readily applied to the part through the instrument, into the eye of which the diseased tissue is by a little management easily engaged.

How often will it be necessary to apply the acid? The answer to this question will depend upon the nature of each case. Where there is only one vascular tumour, or a limited amount of disease, one application, pretty freely made, will suffice; but in cases where there are several tumours or points of disease, as many operations will be needful.

It is necessary for me to say a few words regarding the amount of suffering produced by the application of the nitric acid. Most persons naturally connect *pain* in their imagination with the use of any caustic, arguing from the effects of the agent on the integument. Doubtless, the various caustics which are used cannot be applied to the skin without causing much suffering; but it is far otherwise with the mucous membrane, especially that of the rectum. The general and immediate effect of the acid in most cases, is to cause merely a slight smarting or warmth, which goes off very speedily. In some instances, actual pain of a somewhat severe character is produced, especially when the surface touched is close upon the verge of the anus. There are however instances of hæmorrhoids and prolapsus of long standing, where the parts have become so insensible, that the patients actually do not know when the acid is applied. The reason why I prefer applying it through the speculum is, that the proceeding is perfectly painless, patients having asked me the question whether the acid has been applied or not when the operation is quite finished. It is however a very different matter if any portion of the caustic comes in contact with the sensitive skin of the anus. Should such occur, the pain will be very severe, and will last for hours; hence the obvious necessity of taking the utmost precautions against this.

I can truly say that it has never occurred to me to witness anything like a fatal, or even a dangerous result, after having had a large experience of this remedy. In one case of a patient, who was most anxious to be cured by one operation, I applied the nitric acid much more freely than usual, and produced great suffering for two or three days, with the effect, however, of making a good cure. In another instance, I heard, but was not a witness of the fact, that copious bleeding followed the use of the acid. In a third instance, which occurred very lately, a young lady was treated with the nitric acid for a florid pile. Severe and unaccountable suffering was produced for many days. On making a careful examination, at the end of this period, I discovered a small ulcer, situated at the posterior verge of the anus, and exquisitely painful; suitable remedies relieved the pain in a few hours. On inquiring more minutely into the particulars of this case, I have reasons for believing that this ulcer existed before I applied the acid, and that some of the caustic came into contact with the sore, and produced the most severe suffering. The existence of a painful ulcer or fissure, in conjunction with hæmorrhoidal tumours, is not unfrequent; and an examination, with the view of ascertaining this point, should be instituted, especially if it is found that the patient complains of more than usually severe pain, when at the closet, and lasting for some time subsequently. It is needless to mention that the application of the nitric acid to the rectum when this does exist, must not be thought of.

I have now and then met with cases where retention of urine, and pretty smart bleeding, have occurred after the free use of the nitric acid, but never sufficient to cause me anxiety, and they are symptoms which are easily met.

It is not necessary to confine patients to their bed after the acid has been applied, and this is one of the reasons why the remedy is so desirable, many patients having neither the time nor inclination to submit to an operation which may keep them from their business or pleasures for a fortnight or more.

Having explained the action of this remedy, and the means of applying it, I shall transcribe some illustrative cases, as detailed in my note-book :

CASE V.—Miss B—, aged about forty, consulted me in April, 1854. She was suffering dreadfully with hæmorrhoids, which had existed for more than twelve months. Her symptoms were great irritability of bladder and incontinence of urine; also excessive pain in the lumbar region, and altogether great distress.

On examination, I found a mass of what appeared to be external piles protruding from the anus, and internal to the sphincter were two large vascular tumours. It was one of those cases where a combined operation was necessary—viz., the application of nitric acid to the inner vascular tumours, and the removal of the external ones with the scissors. I ordered her a purgative, and desired her to sit over hot water before my arrival next day, when, finding the parts well protruded, I applied the strong nitric acid to the two inner tumours, and at the same time cut away nearly the whole of the external mass; of course, as I used the scissors at the same time, the patient was compelled to lie in bed, therefore I applied the acid very freely. No evil results followed its use, and on examining her at the end of a week, the internal tumours had nearly disappeared, and that symptom which was so distressing to her—namely, the incontinence of urine—had entirely left her.

In this case, which was a severe instance of

internal piles, accompanied with external protrusion, I performed the two operations of applying nitric acid and removing the external tumours on the same day. I never adopt this proceeding now, believing it to be much better to destroy the internal disease first, and subsequently to cut away any external growth.

CASE VI.—Mr. T—, aged sixty-five, consulted me in May, 1854. Has suffered from hæmorrhoids upwards of twenty years, to such an extent that his comfort has been greatly interfered with; every time he went to the closet the piles came down, and sometimes to such an extent that he could fill the hollow of his hand with them when he passed them up. There was also a great deal of bleeding, and sometimes so much that his drawers were quite saturated, so that he dared not walk out. Of late, however, this excessive hæmorrhage has not troubled him.

On examination, I discovered several large loose folds of integument around the anus, and within their circumference were seen several bright vascular masses of internal piles. I applied the strong nitric acid to one of these tumours lightly, the pain was not severe, and only of short duration, and on his next visit he stated that there had been less protrusion; I therefore used the acid on four other occasions, without giving the patient any distress, and after the fifth operation, finding that the tumours were nearly destroyed, I removed the external growths with the scissors on a separate occasion. These wounds healed rapidly, and in about a week from this date the patient considered himself perfectly cured, not being annoyed by any bleeding, or by any protrusion at the anus whilst at the closet or during walking.

I met this gentleman, quite accidentally, nearly four years

after this treatment had been pursued; he assured me that the cure remained a perfect one.

I have mentioned before that a patient may entirely get rid of his disease by one application, if he will insist upon undergoing the necessary pain and confinement; but it must be used very freely, and a corresponding amount of suffering must be expected.

CASE VII.—Mr. F—, aged about forty, consulted me, in May, 1854. He had suffered for many years from very painful protrusion of the mucous membrane of the rectum. was much distressed by his complaint, and I was requested by the late Dr. Stolworthy to examine this gentleman, and do what operation I considered necessary. On examination, I discovered a very large internal tumour, of a dark bluish colour, mainly consisting of venous texture, and therefore not a kind of case to which I would generally recommend the acid. The affection was, however, the source of vast annoyance, and as the patient was a very irritable subject, and anxious to get cured by one operation, I determined to make him lie in bed, and to use the acid freely.

Accordingly, on the 14th, we obtained some of the fuming nitrous acid, and applied it very freely over the whole diseased surface; the effect of this application was intense pain, which lasted the whole night, and to some degree for the next two or three days; but on the first occasion he had to evacuate the bowels there was no protrusion, and none afterwards; the one application had completely destroyed the disease. I met this gentleman some time afterwards, and he told me he had continued quite well.

It is extraordinary to what an extent some

patients will suffer from this affection, from fear of undergoing the operation by cutting, or by the ligature, and from ignorance of any other means of cure. Sometimes we shall meet with patients who have worn bandages or pessaries for many years. Not long since I met with a gentleman who goes about with a protrusion as large as my fist, which he keeps up with a pessary. He consulted me for another complaint, spoke to me of his hæmorrhoids, but would not submit to any operation. Many such cases may either be cured or materially relieved.

CASE VIII.—Mr. G—, aged forty-five, consulted me, May, 1857. He has had great trouble from piles and protrusion for ten or twelve years, and of late they have become so much worse that he has worn a bandage for three or four years to keep the parts in position, otherwise they generally come down whilst he is walking. On examination, I found that the cause of the protrusion was a large internal pile, not very vascular. I applied the nitrous acid to it.

On the 6th he called to say that he was already much relieved, as on evacuating the bowels he found there was less protrusion. I therefore applied the acid again, and advised him to leave off his bandage. A month afterwards, I had a letter from this gentleman, who was compelled to go into the country before the treatment was finished, and he stated that he had entirely left off the bondage, and had only "a slight inconvenience two or three times, during a little more constipation than otherwise."

In cases of this description it is generally found that the protrusion of the internal hæmorrhoids is owing to, or rather kept up by, the loose folds of thickened integument, which are so often found to be associated with piles. In all such cases it is absolutely necessary to remove these preternatural growths with the scissors; for even where the nitric acid has done its duty well, there will be a tendency in the disease to return if these folds are not excised. I have reason to believe also, that in some of those cases where there is a return of the disease after the application of the ligature, the surgeon has neglected this most essential portion of his work.

I have described a condition of the rectum where there is a general vascular state rather than any distinct tumour, and where the most prominent symptom is hæmorrhage. This is sometimes so excessively severe as to produce an alarming effect upon the patient's health, rendering him or her pale and languid, and incapable of the ordinary duties of life; and even when the bleeding is not sufficient to produce any serious symptoms, it is a source of the utmost annoyance; for this hæmorrhagic condition of the gut the nitric acid is an admirable remedy, and especially if there be any distinct vascular mass from whence the bleeding comes.

CASE IX.—Mr. C—, aged twenty-nine, sent to me by Dr. Beaman, October 6th, 1857. He had been troubled with "piles" for two years, which had given him more or less trouble; but during the last six months there has been a considerable amount of bleeding every day; this has been increased in a great degree by violent horse-exercise, this gentleman being very fond of hunting. The hæmorrhage is the symptom for which he sought advice, although there has been some protrusion when at stool. On examination, I found the mucous membrane of the rectum in an unhealthy and congested state, and at one point a distinct vascular mass. I advised him to take a full dose of castor-oil on the evening of the 7th, and to come to me on the following morning. On that day, finding the mucous membrane and the vascular mass well protruded, I touched it with strong nitric acid freely. Next day he sent for me; I found him in bed, in considerable pain, the diseased surface having protruded, and the integuments being considerably swollen. I recommended him to lie in bed for a few hours, and ordered hot fomentations. In the evening I found him up, free from pain.

13th.—This patient has been in the country, has scarcely any bleeding; he had taken some castor-oil the previous night, which had brought the bowel down, so I applied the acid again.

15th.—Applied the acid again.

20th.—This patient scarcely complains of anything except a slight bleeding. On examination with the speculum, I found a portion of the mucous membrane in a vascular condition, and I touched it freely with nitric acid.

24th.—There is no protrusion, and only slight bleeding. I examined him again with the speculum, and applied the acid to the vascular spot. He did not even know when I was touching the part with the nitric acid, so painless was the application when used through the speculum. I saw this patient again in a few days, and wrote for him an injection containing sulphate of iron, to be used if needful.

This patient consulted me several months afterwards for another complaint, told me that he had hunted much through the season, and had not any bleeding since he left me, nor had he been compelled at any time to use the astringent lotion.

I have already stated that I would not recommend the nitric acid in those cases of hæmorrhoids of long standing where there are several distinct tumours of considerable size, and where, from continual irritation, they have become indurated, are not in a great degree vascular, and do not bleed. In such instances, I believe it is better that the ligature should be applied, as disappointment would probably ensue, and discredit be brought upon a remedy which is so useful in proper cases. It will, however, happen that patients suffering from this aggravated form of the disorder will consult the surgeon, and will not undergo the operation of the ligature, but will readily submit to any treatment which may give a fair chance of lessening their sufferings, without producing any risk, or confining them to their bed.

CASE X.—Mr. G—, aged fifty-six, in weak health, consulted me May 12th. He has had piles for fifteen years, and some time since he consulted a surgeon, who recommended him to wear a pessary, which gave him some relief. During the last three years he has become much worse, the diseased parts protruding not only when at the closet, but even when he walks about. There never has been much bleeding.

I caused him to sit over hot water for some minutes, and then examining him, found a considerable tumour protruded. There were four distinct hæmorrhoidal tumours, two of them being as large as the top of the finger, very much indurated, not vascular, and not painful on pressure; the other two were smaller, more vascular, and evidently of a more recent formation than the others. Outside the sphincter was a quantity of loose and thickened integument. On the inner aspect of the larger piles the mucous membrane was thinner, somewhat abraded, and more vascular.

This case was evidently not a promising one for treatment by nitric acid; but the patient had heard of this remedy, and asked me if I could hold out any chance of relief by its means. I strongly recommended the ligature, but, on his asking the question, was obliged to tell him that this operation was not without danger. He preferred the chance of relief by the acid. The parts being well protruded, I applied the acid to the inner portion of the two large hæmorrhoidal tumours. This application was done at my own house; it gave the patient hardly any pain, and he rode home afterwards in his carriage.

14th.—He has not had any pain since the application of the acid, and there has been much less protrusion. On causing him to sit over hot water, it was difficult to get more than half what was prolapsed before. One of the large piles, however, came into view, and I touched that with the nitric acid, also one of the smaller tumours.

17th.—This gentleman has not suffered any protrusion when at the closet, and has informed me that he stood for upwards of two hours together to-day witnessing an exhibition, and that afterwards there was not any protrusion, which would most assuredly have been the case before he consulted me. As there would be some difficulty in his protruding the parts, I introduced the speculum, and applied the acid through it to one of the tumours. This application caused more smarting than any of the others.

20th.—He has suffered considerable inconvenience, but no pain since the last application; this has now gone off. He states that he is so much improved, that when he goes to the closet the piles no longer protrude. I, however, made another examination with the speculum, and applied the acid to a portion of the disease which came into view. This application the patient literally did not feel. He is going into the country well pleased with the benefit he has obtained, and has promised to come again and see me if there be any further protrusion. I have strongly advised him to allow me to remove the loose skin from around the anus; having explained to him that in all probability if this be left it will increase, and tend to produce some further prolapsus.

This case is of necessity somewhat incomplete, but it is an instructive one, because it shows that even in those cases where the ligature is imperatively called for, apparently great relief, if not an actual cure, may be brought about by the judicious application of the nitric acid. It also illustrated another point which I have already alluded to, viz., the advantage in possessing some means which will supplant the ligature in cases where patients, either from dread or from an unwillingness to lie up, will not undergo that process, and will prefer to suffer from the pain and inconvenience of their disorder, rather than submit to the ordeal proposed; whereas, on a candid explanation of the little suffering produced by the nitric acid, and its mode of action, they will gladly take advantage of such a remedy.

CASE XL.—Mr. W—, aged thirty, consulted me March 17th, 1858. He has been a delicate man always, and has suffered for the last four years from disease of the rectum, first showing itself by pain and bleeding. For the last two years he has never had a motion without losing much blood. He has been accustomed to hunt a great deal, and on his return, after a day's sport, he has found his small-clothes saturated with blood. His countenance indicated loss of blood, his face being very pallid and pasty.

On examination, I discovered that the anus was surrounded by several large excrescences of a pendulous nature; and, internally, the mucous membrane of the rectum was in a very diseased condition, there being on either side hæmorrhoidal tumours of considerable size, very vascular, and covered with a very thick and diseased membrane. Bleeding was produced by this examination. It is only latterly that this gentleman has been much annoyed by protrusion; but so great has this become, that sometimes the gut has kept down for thirty hours at a time after an evacuation.

I explained to this gentleman that his case was one well adapted for a combined operation, that it would be necessary to cut off the external growths, and then attack the internal mischief by some other means; and, as the hæmorrhagic character was chiefly marked, I advised the application of strong nitric acid to the mucous membrane.

On the 18th I removed the pendulous growths with the scissors, and on the 21st I applied the strong nitric acid to the diseased mucous membrane. This application was not attended or followed by much pain; and on the 25th, finding the diseased surface much reduced, I applied it again. On the 29th, as there still remained a small portion of diseased mucous membrane, I made a third and last application. After this the bleeding and protrusion ceased, and the patient returned home.

This patient was confined to his bed for some days, because the use of the scissors was followed by considerable bleeding, and retention of urine.

I had the gratification of seeing this gentleman walk into my house on the 13th of November, just eight months after he had left my care. He was looking remarkably stout and well, and told me that, although he had hunted much, he had not had the slightest return of the bleeding or protrusion.

There are some exceedingly severe cases of internal hæmorrhoids which produce so much suffering, and are attended with such a large amount of bleeding, that the general health is reduced to a very low verge, and the most prudent course to adopt in such cases is to employ the remedy upon which the most dependence can be placed, viz., the ligature, but the condition of the health may be such as to prevent this treatment, or the patient will not be persuaded to undergo it. It is then that nitric acid may be substituted, especially if the tumours present the bright red vascular appearance before mentioned; and, if the mucous membrane is not indurated, the hæmorrhoidal tumours may be of large size, and have existed so many years, that a perfect cure cannot be brought about by the treatment in question; but such a vast amount of relief is given, that the patient may be, in one sense, considered as cured.

CASE XII.—Miss O—, aged thirty-eight, consulted me February 18th, 1859. The first symptoms of her complaint appeared five years previously, when she had hæmorrhage and protrusion of the bowel whilst at the closet. These symptoms degenerated into a severe attack, which confined her to bed for several weeks. After having partially recovered from this, she suffered more or less from both bleeding and protrusion, and her health suffered severely. The immediate cause of her applying to me was the circumstance of constant bleeding having taken place from the bowel, not only whilst she was at the closet, but even when she was quiet.

On examination, I found a considerable mass at the anus,

consisting externally of long folds of thickened and loose skin, and internally of two large hæmorrhoidal tumours of a bright red colour, and having the mucous membrane slightly ulcerated. These tumours presented themselves, without any effort, on the part of the patient. On examition of the rectum higher up with the speculum, I found the mucous membrane generally in a very vascular and thickened state. Her general health was in a wretched condition, her face was pale and bloodless, and there was an amount of muscular debility, that amounted almost to palsy. There was also that extreme and continued headache, which is such a certain accompaniment of continued and profuse bleeding.

Now, this was a case where it would, perhaps, have been best to employ the ligature, but the health was reduced, and there were other circumstances which rendered it inexpedient, so that I thought it right to attempt to arrest the bleeding, and destroy the vascular tumours with nitric acid. I, therefore, applied the acid to a portion of the diseased tissue.

22nd.—Considerable pain and bleeding followed this application; but there has been less descent of the hæmorrhoids. I used the acid again.

Much less pain followed the last application, but there was more bleeding when at the closet. The part does not protrude half so much as it did, and the patient assures me she can return it without any trouble. On examination I found much less protrusion. I applied the acid through the speculum.

March 1st.—Still less protrusion; applied the acid through the speculum.

7th.—The bowel has not been down for three days, since the 4th, when I used the acid. The bleeding, although it has been much less, has not yet been arrested. I have, therefore, ordered her to throw up the sulphate of iron injection daily.

18th.—This patient called on me to-day. There has not been any bleeding for several days, and no protrusion. I recommended that she should have the pendulous flaps of thickened skin removed from around the anus. I effected this operation with the scissors.

31st.—The wounds made by the scissors are just healed. There has not been the slightest bleeding since the last report, and only on one occasion, when the bowels had been evacuated by medicine, was there any protrusion. Her general health was improved. I recommended her to continue the use of the iron lotion, and to take the confection of senna every other night.

This was one of the most severe cases for which I have used the nitric acid with such great relief. As I have before stated, had circumstances admitted it, it would have been better to have employed the ligature at once, because the effects produced by the disease were of such a nature as to preclude any treatment which might be doubtful; but I had no hesitation in telling this patient that the nitric acid would give her immense relief, and the result justified my recommendation. It is likely enough that, at some future time, this patient may suffer somewhat from bleeding, and some slight protrusion; but, should either of these symptoms take place, I doubt not that they would be remedied by the nitric acid in a very speedy manner. It has been noticed, that at the end of the treatment of this case, I removed, with the scissors, the loose folds of thickened integument from around the margin of the anus. This step is an important one after most of the operations for internal hæmorrhoids. If there is a great redundancy of skin in a diseased condition, and this is left, the chances are very great, that it will cause further descent of the bowel at some future time. The removal of it by the knife or scissors, and the subsequent cicatrization which takes place, produces a certain amount of contraction, and bracing up of the parts, which acts most beneficially in preventing a return of the disease. Of course, it is necessary to be careful in avoiding the too free use of the scissors; for, if too much integument be taken away, great contraction might take place.

The following case illustrates the beneficial effects of nitric acid, even in a case to which, from the structure of the diseased parts, the treatment would not appear to be particularly applicable:

CASE XIII.—Mr. M—, aged forty, from Canada, consulted me August 6th, 1859. He had suffered from internal hæmorrhoids for seven years. The first symptom was severe hæmorrhage, which, a year after, became followed by protrusion whilst he was at the closet. The protruded parts became larger in size, and gradually produced increased annoyance, but the bleeding ceased. During the last five years the patient has not had a motion without the piles protruding; and if he went to the closet in the morning, the parts remained protruded all the day. To prevent this, he has latterly got into the habit of visiting the closet at nighttime, so that the bowel goes back on retiring to bed. There is frequently a protrusion even when he is walking.

On examination, I found a very considerable protrusion, consisting, on the right side, of two or three distinct hæmorrhoidal tumours of a deep blue, venous character. On the left side, there was a portion of prolapsed mucous membrane, about the size of the top of my thumb, and but little altered from its natural appearance. Externally, there was a redundancy of loose and thickened integument. The patient was in pretty good health, but pale and spiritless.

I informed this gentleman that the ligature of the hæmorrhoidal tumours would be the most certain treatment, and that I could not confidently recommend the use of anything else; but, as there was no doubt that the prolapsed portion of mucous membrane might be successfully treated by nitric acid, it was possible great benefit might result from the use of this agent. His time for staying in England being limited, he wished me to try the nitric acid.

I therefore applied the acid to the prolapsed part very freely. Its use was attended with only a little smarting.

8th.—As he walked away from my house the bowel unfortunately protruded, and the patient could not return it by his own efforts; and he has suffered a good deal of pain from the parts being gripped by the sphincter. On examination, I found the protruded bowel in a semi-sloughy condition. I applied the acid again, and returned the protruded parts with great care. The manipulation necessary for this purpose produced great pain.

13th.—This gentleman came to me to-day in very good spirits, telling me that his bowels had been moved three times within the last forty-eight hours, and that there has not been any protrusion whatever.

16th.—He called to-day, and informed me that he has evacuated the bowels regularly every morning since his last visit to me, and that he has no protrusion whatever. On examination, I could not discover a trace of his disease; but there was a small external pile posteriorly, which I snipped off with scissors. This gentleman called on me in the summer of 1861, and told me he had remained quite well.

I scarcely expected that this patient would get such a very speedy and decided cure, for the hæmorrhoidal tumours were of that nature for which I do not generally apply the nitric acid; but the action of the agent on the prolapsed portion of mucous membrane was most successful; and, moreover, the removal of the disease was doubtless much assisted by the strangulating effect of the sphincter ani on the whole mass, which was as it were accidentally kept up for some hours. This circumstance shows how necessary it is to return the bowel thoroughly after the application of the acid; for the protrusion is very liable to come down as soon as the patient moves about, unless the parts are well put back. For this reason, I prefer making the first application of the acid at the patient's own house, so that he or she may keep quiet for an hour or two afterwards, and thus prevent the possibility of a descent of the tumours.

In the next cases are seen illustrations of the good effects of nitric acid, in severe instances of internal piles, attended by hæmorrhage.

CASE XIV.—Mr. C—, aged twenty-three, sent to me by Dr. Beaman, May 21st. He informed me that he had been subject to internal piles for three years; they always protruded considerably when he was at the closet during the last few months, and sometimes they have come down when he has been walking. The most serious symptom however has been bleeding of a very profuse character, which has rendered him very weak. He complained much of debility and shortness of breath, and his face presented that pallid aspect which so distinctly denotes great, or long continued, loss of blood.

On examining the rectum, I discovered that the mucous membrane of the lower part of the bowel was in an unhealthy condition, and on the right side there was protruded, without any effort on the part of the patient, a large, florid, vascular, pile, without any distinct base. It was just the case for the use of the nitric acid—so I applied it carefully to the hæmorrhoidal tumour.

25th.—Bleeding continues, perhaps, to a greater extent, and there is still protrusion. I applied the acid again very carefully.

28th.—This gentleman suffered considerably, for a few hours, from the last application, but he is considerably better, there is scarcely any protrusion.

June 1st.—Bleeding has almost entirely ceased, and there is no protrusion. I applied the acid again.

10th.—The patient came to-day, saying that he felt quite well, and that he has not had any protrusion at all, and that only once since I saw him was there any hæmorrhage, which was very slight when he was at the closet.

CASE XV.—Mr. Alder Fisher, in December, 1859, asked me to see a young lady, aged twenty-two, who was suffering severely from bleeding. On examination I found a protrusion of not large size, and a very congested state of the lower part of the rectum altogether. The mucous membrane covering the protruded part was smooth and healthy. This lady had suffered for more than a year from hæmorrhage, which at times was very violent, and recently she had had a prolonged attack, which had told upon her system, rendering her pallid and feeble.

On the 13th, having first emptied the rectum by an injection, and having got the mucous membrane well prolapsed, I carefully applied the nitric acid to the whole of the portion which generally protruded, and also to the remaining part of the mucous lining of the lower part of the gut which was now brought into view, and was found to be granular and very vascular. As the application was a severe one, I advised her to keep her bed, and ordered an opiate.

16th.—The bowels have been acted upon by castor-oil, with some bleeding, but no protrusion. I introduced the speculum, and applied the nitric acid to a part which had not been touched.

19th—Finding no trace of protrusion, I removed some external folds of loose skin from the anus.

29th.—She has had an evacuation without medicine, free

from pain or protrusion, and with only trifling bleeding. In a fortnight this lady went to France.

In March, 1862, I had a letter from this patient, in which she informed me, that for some little time after the treatment had been adopted she suffered from the same symptoms, yet, as time went on, they gradually and completely left her, and she expressed herself much gratified with the results of the method used for her relief.

I have witnessed the most extraordinary relief of symptoms of long standing by one or two applications of nitric acid, more especially of hæmorrhage, but I am not aware that I have ever met with an instance where the remedy acted with more success than in the following. The case also serves to illustrate the particular morbid condition for which the nitric acid is so admirably adapted.

CASE XVI.—Mr. H—, aged forty, sent to me by Mr. West, of Westminster, August 9th, 1860. He informed me that he had suffered from piles for twenty years, that during the last few years the tumours have protruded every time he visited the closet, and there has been bleeding daily. His appearance did not belie his statement, for his face was pale and his lips bloodless; latterly, also, he had complained much of indigestion.

On examination, I found several small hæmorrhoidal tumours protruding at the anus. They were extremely vascular, and of a bright scarlet colour. I applied the nitric acid very carefully to the parts, and the patient walked home from my house.

14th.—He came to me to-day, saying he was better than he had been for twenty years. His bowels have been acted upon with scarcely any pain, protrusion, or bleeding. On examination, there is no trace of the disease visible; so I introduced a speculum and applied nitric acid to a vascular portion of the mucous membrane.

20th.—This patient visited me to-day, and it was extraordinary to witness the improvement in his appearance. He stated that he was quite free from any symptoms. I have not seen him since, as most probably would have been the case, had he been further troubled.

I have stated that the nitric acid is not suitable for those cases where the hæmorrhoidal tumours are of a dark-blue colour, and chiefly composed of veins. If it is applied in such cases the surgeon will generally be disappointed. Should, however, this condition be accompanied by severe hæmorrhage, the nitric acid may act most beneficially. The following case illustrates this well, and may be contrasted with the one just narrated:

CASE XVII.—Mr. M—, aged twenty-five, consulted me in May, 1860. He had the aspect of a man who had lost much blood, and he informed me that for several years he had suffered with bleeding piles. At times the loss of blood had been great, and he had suffered excessively.

On examination, I found the whole mucous membrane of the lower part of the rectum in a very unhealthy condition, it being very vascular, thickened, and of a deep livid colour, there were also several varices of the same colour within the anus, and throwing out a considerable quantity of blood. Although I could not promise this gentleman that the remedy would be attended with success, I thought it worth a trial, and accordingly applied it carefully, and repeated it twice more within the next fortnight. A week after the third application, this gentleman called upon me to say that he was free from bleeding, and had scarcely any protrusion. In November he called to say he was quite free from all inconvenience; he had improved vastly in health and appearance. In March, 1862, I accidentally met this patient in the street; he was in robust health, and all he experienced of his former symptoms was an occasional slight bleeding on unusual exertion.

I do not think it necessary to give any further illustrations of the use of nitric acid in internal hæmorrhoids, but there are one or two points on which information may be sought; and the first is, as regards the want of success which has attended its use. It would be absurd, of course, to maintain that the nitric acid will cure or relieve all cases of internal piles. So uncertain is the practice of medicine, and even of surgery, that success cannot always be depended on, even when we bring to bear the greatest skill and utmost care in the use of remedies, and it is only quacks, cancer-curers, et id genus omne, who will assume infallibility for their remedies. The nitric acid will sometimes fail in doing good, and I am willing to admit that it has disappointed me; but this has been the case in only a few instances—and even in those I believe that this disappointment arose either from a want of judgment on my part, or from an improper application of the remedy. As I become more and more careful in the selection of the cases, it is my belief that the disappointments as to results will be very rare.

Since these remarks were written for the last edition of this work, I have had extensive opportunities of employing the nitric acid for internal hæmorrhoids, and of testing the value of this agent, and, although I have resorted to the ligature more frequently than was my custom, I still find that a considerable proportion of the cases which are submitted to my notice can be benefited or cured by the careful application of the acid. Nevertheless, I am bound to state that the objection brought against this agent, that it is an uncertain one, is to some extent valid, and that in a few cases where it has been employed by myself with the greatest care, scarcely more than a trifling effect has been produced. I must, however, admit that the failures when they have occurred have resulted from my want of care in the selection of cases. I have used it occasionally in instances where the hæmorrhoidal tumours have been large, and where the disease had existed so long that the mucous membrane had become thickened and had lost its vascularity. It is true that in such cases the attempts to cure were chiefly induced by the urgent representations of the patient, and that I had given a cautious opinion with reference to the result.

On the other hand, it has occurred to me to meet with cases where, from my previous experience, I should have been led to consider the remedy useless, and yet, to my great surprise, a few applications have been followed by the most gratifying results.

My opinion has undergone no change with respect to the value and efficacy of nitric acid when employed in well selected cases, such as have been alluded to, in some of these instances, especially where hæmorrhage has been the most prominent feature, the result of one or two applications of the acid alone has been marvellous. With respect to the permanency of the cure, in several instances, both of hæmorrhoids and prolapsus, where the agent has been employed, I have been able to ascertain that the result has been permanent in some, whilst in others there has been some slight and temporary return of symptoms readily removed by a resort to the remedy. I generally guard against any misunderstanding with a patient on this point, by stating the possibility of a return of some of the symptoms at a future period, after apparently the most successful results have been produced, at the same time giving the assurance that, should any symptom such as bleeding recur, it will be readily put a stop to by an application of the nitric acid.

I must here say a few additional words regarding the pain attending the use of the nitric acid, especially as I find there is an impression, both amongst patients and medical men, that the use of nitric acid is of necessity accompanied with great pain; nothing is more erroneous, for in by far the majority of cases where the acid is used to the mucous membrane of the rectum alone, the patient complains of a slight burning sensation only, or of no pain whatever. Several persons have told me that they actually could not tell if I had used it or not. I have met with a case now and then, since the last edition of this book was written, in which the patient suffered somewhat severely; but when this has been so, either the mucous membrane to which the acid has been applied was close to the verge of the anus, or a portion of the acid has, through my carelessness, come into contact with the integument.

When there is a doubt about the case as regards the applicability of the nitric acid, and the patient is not a fit subject for the ligature, or will not submit to this operation, I adopt the course of treatment suggested originally, if I am not mistaken, by the late Mr. Cusack, and recommended by Mr. Lee. This consists in compressing the hæmorrhoidal tumour by means of a blunt pair of scissors or clamp, and snipping away the free portion with sharp scissors; the cut surface of the tumour is then carefully wiped with a piece of sponge or lint, and then the nitric acid is freely applied to every portion. Of course, no bleeding can take place, if the base of the hæmorrhoid be well secured by the clamp; and so soon as the raw surface is thoroughly imbued with the acid, the clamp is removed, and although the pressure is taken off, bleeding is arrested by the action of the caustic.

This is an excellent mode of treatment for those cases which cannot be cured by nitric acid alone, and even in cases where this agent alone will suffice, it may be recommended; for it is more certain in its results, and only one operation is necessary. The pain is trifling, and the danger can be deemed scarcely greater than that attending the simple use of the acid, if due precautions be taken to prevent bleeding, which may be effected by not hurrying the process and by attending to various details. Thus, it should be seen that the clamp be well brought home, and the tumour be thoroughly compressed, and held so by an assistant before the sharp scissors are used. After the acid has been applied, the base of the tumour should be compressed for about five minutes before it is set free; and when the clamp is removed, it should be effected gradually, so that if any bleeding should take place, it may be readily detected, and a further application of the acid be made. If bleeding goes on notwithstanding this, either the actual cautery may be applied, or a thread may be cast around the base of the tumour whilst it is still compressed, and all bleeding will be effectually stopped. On one occasion, I was troubled a great deal by bleeding during this operation. I had snipped away an extensive portion of mucous membrane, and applied the acid, and was about to remove the clamp slowly, when I found that blood was issuing very freely from the surface of the divided and cauterized portion. A further application of the acid did not quite arrest it; therefore I tied a ligature around the base of the bleeding part, and no further hæmorrhage occurred.

I shall defer the relation of cases treated in this manner until I come to the subject of Prolapsus of the Rectum, to which affection it is also particularly well adapted, and in which it is employed exactly in the same way. In that portion of the work will be found details of cases where hæmorrhoidal tumours and prolapsus of the rectum were successfully treated by the combined method of the clamp and nitric acid.

I was taken to task by a reviewer of my

last edition for not having said anything about the treatment of internal hæmorrhoids by the écraseur. Doubtless, I was as well acquainted as my critic with the instrument in question, and with the various uses to which it had been applied. I had not been unmindful that the écraseur had been somewhat extensively employed for the removal of hæmorrhoidal tumours, but I was unable to recognise the superiority, or even the prudence of such a mode of treatment, seeing that we possessed two such admirable remedial measures in the shape of the ligature and the use of nitric acid; and therefore I said nothing about this new instrument. My silence has been amply justified by the information which has been recently afforded us; for in the 'Lancet' for November 10th, 1860, I find it stated that the operation for the removal of hæmorrhoidal tumours by the écraseur had been followed in several instances by stricture of the rectum. Since this announcement, we have heard little or nothing of the same hazardous and unscientific mode of treatment; and I can only congratulate myself that I was not induced, by the glowing reports of successful cases, to recommend a practice which would be productive of such serious mischief. One of the great advantages supposed to belong to the use of the écraseur was, that the hæmorrhoidal tumours could be removed without the occurrence of bleeding. But a short time since, however, I saw a case where the écraseur had been used for the removal of internal piles by a well-known surgeon, a few days previously. I noticed that the patient was exceedingly blanched, and on inquiry I ascertained that a most profuse bleeding had occurred a few hours after the operation had been completed, and when it was supposed that all dread of this event had passed by.

PROLAPSUS OF THE RECTUM.

During the time that the rectum is evacuating its contents in a natural and normal manner, more or less extrusion of the mucous membrane occurs, but this is only momentarily. The part is immediately withdrawn within the anal orifice, and no inconvenience results. When however from some particular cause, there is any impediment to the return of this membrane, those changes which ultimately lead to the disease we are considering occur; the mucous membrane becomes congested and swollen, its attachment to the muscular tissue, naturally loose, is weakened, and in course of time the protrusion of the membrane becomes habitual—constituting one form of prolapsus of the rectum, and that the most frequent.

In other cases however, there is a protrusion, not only of the mucous and sub-mucous tissues, but of the whole of the thickness of the lower part of the bowel as well. A preparation in the Museum of King's College puts an end to all doubt on this point. This kind of prolapsus occurs not unfrequently in children, and is of very great extent, sometimes the protruded bowel being five or six inches in length. In very old people this complete prolapsus of the rectum occurs, reaching to an unusual size. On examining a recent case of prolapsus of the rectum, where the least amount of change has taken place in the structure of the parts, as for instance, in a child, the protruded part forms a tumour of an oblong shape and cylindrical form, presenting externally the smooth vascular surface of the mucous membrane, which is generally more or less of a bright red colour, and covered with mucus; at the extremity of the tumour is the orifice or cavity of the bowel, and at the anus there is no deep furrow between it and the protruded part, as there is in intussusception of the rectum. In the adult even, when the prolapse is large and of recent occurrence, the mucous membrane may be as unchanged in appearance and texture as when it occurs in the child, but the tumour has more of a globular form.

The most frequent condition however in which a prolapsus of the rectum is seen, is where there are one or two lateral folds of the membrane varying from one to two inches in length, protruded from the anus, or one unbroken ring of protruded membrane is seen, but this is more rare. If the disease has not long existed, the membrane is not much changed in appearance, being only somewhat thickened and more vascular than natural: but should the bowel have been habitually prolapsed for some years, considerable changes take place, and on examining an old case the following will be the appearances: Externally, there will be a ring of thickened and congested integument; within this the flaps of mucous membrane hang down, their lower portions being much thickened, having lost the peculiar character of mucous membrane, and assimilated to integument; this change has taken place in this part because the most dependent portion is that which either habitually remains protruded altogether, or is protruded for a longer time and more exposed. On separating the flaps of the prolapsus, the upper part of the membrane is found either but little altered from its natural character, being red, smooth and vascular, or superficial ulceration may have taken place where the two portions have been in contact. There is more or less mucous discharge produced, but in pure prolapsus there is little hæmorrhage.

Sometimes in persons advanced in life, the protruded part forms a tumour as large as the fist or larger, which has habitually protruded for a long time. In such a case a very large proportion of the tumour consists of membrane, more like leather than the natural tissue. In these old standing cases, the sphincter becomes extremely relaxed and the anus very capacious; there is generally a redundancy of loose and thickened skin around. Sometimes it hangs down in long pendulous flaps; this state of the parts adds materially to the facility of the occurrence of the prolapsus.

In many cases the prolapsus of the rectum is complicated with distinct hæmorrhoidal tumours, which in fact are mainly if not entirely the originators of the affection; for, when one or more internal tumours exist, they themselves, each time the bowels act, become protruded, and draw portions of the mucous membrane down with them; so that not unfrequently a patient presents himself with one or more folds of prolapsed membrane, and at the same time with distinct hæmorrhoidal tumours.

The inconvenience and suffering which prolapsus causes is considerable; for although at the outset of the affection the protruded part may pretty readily return within the sphincter after an evacuation, as time wears on, it becomes necessary for the patient himself to return the part, which is not rarely a task of difficulty, and attended with pain. Moreover, from the contiguity of the rectum to the neck of the bladder and urethra, there is often great distress of these parts; constant irritability and even retention of urine, being an accompaniment of the affection. Pain and uneasiness is also felt in the loins and down the thighs; the intestinal canal and stomach also sympathise, the patient being troubled with flatulence, loss of appetite, and low spirits.

If the prolapsus, which may usually be put back, cannot be returned by the patient, and is allowed to remain, most violent symptoms occur—extreme pain in the part, and retention of urine; and if unsuccessful attempts are made to reduce the swelling, which is in all probability tightly constricted by the sphincter, violent inflammation of the part, attended with severe constitutional suffering occurs; and in some instances sloughing of the protruded bowel takes place, by which means a cure is brought about; but the mischief may be so severe as to cause death. In cases where a prolapsus occurs in children to a great extent, and has been allowed to remain down for two or three days, the local and constitutional changes are not so severe; the prolapsed membrane, however, becomes exceedingly congested.

The causes of prolapsus are constitutional and local: thus, the disease is very frequently met with in individuals who have suffered from general debility and laxity of fibre. In children especially, the affection is met with in instances where the health has been much reduced by insufficient nutriment, bad air, and want of proper attention. An adult or old person who suffers much from prolapsus will have a weak pulse, a flabby tongue, and impaired digestion;

and a child presents an unhealthy and dry skin, a foul tongue, and a tumid belly. The local causes which produce falling of the bowel in children are stone in the bladder and ascarides. In adults, constipation, sedentary occupation, the straining caused by stricture of the urethra, and enlargement of the prostate are fertile causes of the disease. There is no doubt, moreover, that the pernicious plan of frequently using copious enemata is very constantly productive of the disorder.

In considering the treatment for prolapsus of the rectum, we shall first refer to that which is necessary in removing the affection as it is met with in young children. In the first place, it is necessary to seek for the cause. And especial inquiry should be made with reference to the urinary apparatus; for it not unfrequently happens that it is the irritation of a calculus in the bladder which produces the extrusion of the gut; and if this be so, it is obvious that the only remedy consists in the removal of the stone. If there be not stone in the bladder, a collection of ascarides in the rectum may originate the disease; and the destruction of these parasites by a few doses of scammony and calomel, together with the daily injection of a few ounces of strong infusion of quassia, will prevent the disease.

In by far the larger proportion of cases occurring in children, the general health will be found to be at fault, and this must be attended to before the prolapsus can be got rid of. In the first place it is necessary to return the protruded bowel; and this is sometimes a work of difficulty, because the child struggles violently and cries. The protruded bowel should be gently but firmly grasped by the right hand, well oiled; careful pressure, so as to empty the vessels, should be employed, until the whole be returned within the sphincter. When the protrusion has been large, however, and the child is very violent, the gut will soon fall again; and in this case the best plan to pursue is to place the child under the influence of chloroform, and the bowel will then be readily returned. A pad and bandage should then be employed, in order to secure the part. The secretions of the liver and bowels should be rendered healthy by the use of small doses of rhubarb and Hydr. cum Creta, the skin be kept in good order by the warm bath; the child should be carried about in the fresh air, the diet must be nutritious and in small volume, and the strength and appetite are to be increased by small doses of the Pulvis Cinchonæ and soda. As the health improves the prolapsus will cease to appear; but should this persist, the part may be bathed with a solution of sulphate of iron, gr. j to ℨj of water, or an injection of tincture of sesquichloride of iron ℨj to ℨvj of water may be thrown up every morning after the evacuation of the bowels, and after the protrusion has been returned. In some cases the prolapsus will recur whenever the child evacuates the bowel. This, however, may be prevented by so managing that the child should be in a kneeling posture during the act. Another plan, which sometimes succeeds in preventing the protrusion, consists in an attendant drawing on one side the skin of the anus with some force during the time the bowel is being emptied. By this means a certain amount of temporary contraction is produced, which prevents the descent of the gut.

In adults, a considerable number of the cases which are not severe, and which have not been of long standing, may be cured by careful attention to the removal of those causes which have produced it. Thus, if the affection has resulted from violent straining and constipation of the bowels, some mild aperient should be exhibited occasionally, which will prevent accumulation in the bowels, and render the contents more fluid. The compound rhubarb pill at night will have the effect, or, what is perhaps better, one or two teaspoonfuls of confection of senna should be taken. The patient should not eat largely, and should especially avoid vegetables in any quantity. He should take exercise, and be especially careful to use plenty of cold water to the parts after the action of the bowels. Occasionally a little cold water, or a few ounces of the decoction of oak-bark, may be thrown up the rectum; and if there be the least protrusion after the evacuation of the bowels, the gut, after having first been well sponged, should be carefully returned.

By attention to these various measures, a prolapsus of small extent and not of long standing may either be entirely cured, or may be prevented from increasing or proving troublesome, and therefore it is of the highest importance to place reliance upon medical treatment in such cases. In by far the greater majority of cases, however, which are presented to the notice of the surgeon, the prolapsus is either very extensive, or has existed so long a time that medical treatment will be of no use whatever, and then some strictly surgical means must be adopted, if a cure or even palliation of the disease is looked for. If the case is of only recent occurrence—but the prolapsus is very voluminous and is incapable of being returned, thereby causing much alarm and suffering—it is the duty of the surgeon at once to reduce the prolapsed bowel. This is best effected by placing the patient on his side, with his knees drawn up, and grasping the tumour either with the naked hand, well oiled, or with a cloth intervening. Firm and steady compression should be used until the whole of the tumour be removed within the sphincter. The patient should then lie quiet for some hours, and afterwards a pad should be applied to the anus, and secured by a firm bandage across the perineum and around the loins. In order to prevent a return of the prolapsus, the whole or greater portion of the mucous membrane should be smeared over with solid nitrate of silver, previous to its being returned by the surgeon.

The following case is a good illustration of this plan of treatment:

CASE XVIII.—Called February 21st, by Dr. Wildbore, to see Miss S—, aged eighty-two, who was suffering acutely from prolapsus of the rectum. No distinct history could be learned about the case, but it was supposed that the disease had existed for many years; it was not, however, until the day previous that attention was called to the bowel by the continual desire of the patient to relieve herself. Dr. Wildbore then discovered an immense protrusion of the rectum, which he returned without difficulty; the gut, however, soon protruded again, and the patient could scarcely be kept in bed a minute in consequence of the irritation produced by the descent of the bowel, and although she was in good health for her age, the disease told rapidly upon her.

On examination, I found a large protrusion of the whole thickness of the bowel, the mucous membrane being smooth and velvety. I smeared the whole surface freely over with solid nitrate of silver, and returned the tumour. I found the anus very capacious.

On the 28th I was called again to see this lady, and ascertained that the prolapsus had returned the same day I had returned it, in consequence of her repeated visits to the closet. Dr. Wildbore had, therefore, again applied the nitrate of silver less freely, and returned the tumour. It kept up for two days, when, on her going to empty her bowels, it returned again, but somewhat less in size. I therefore very freely smeared the caustic over the entire mucous surface of the prolapsus again, thoroughly replaced it, and recommended that the patient, who was much exhausted, should keep to the recumbent position entirely, and take as much stimulating nourishment as possible.

This treatment was followed by the best results. On the next action of the bowels, the prolapsus did not return, and a fortnight afterwards I was informed by Dr. Wildbore that the old lady had recovered her health, and had had no sign of prolapse.

In order to bring about an effectual cure of the more chronic and severe cases of prolapsus, more decided means must be adopted. We have seen that the disease essentially consists in a relaxed and thickened condition of the mucous membrane, and a separation as it were of it from the muscular coat, and when this is involved also, a weakness and detachment of the whole of the thickness of the bowel from the surrounding supports. The object to be obtained is to reduce the redundancy or relaxation of the mucous membrane, to promote adhesion between the several tissues composing the bowel, and to brace up the anus and the sphincter. The late Mr. Hey, of Leeds, was the first to propose a proceeding which ensured the latter result, and this consisted in removing the loose and pendulous flaps of skin, which existed around the margin of the anus, in the case alluded to by him in his "Practical Observations on Surgery," p. 443. In some cases where the sphincter is very relaxed, and the flaps of integument very loose and thick, a cure may be brought about by the removal of these alone; but when the prolapsus is very large, and a considerable portion of the mucous membrane has been converted into tissue approaching to integument, it will be necessary to adopt the modification of the operation proposed by Dupuytren, which consists in removing radiating folds, not only of the skin at the margin of the anus, but also of the diseased mucous membrane. The operation is effected by laying hold of the fold of the skin on each side of the anus, with a pair of forceps, then with a sharp pair of scissors curved, and dipping their points as it were into the anus, removing both skin and mucous membrane. In very severe cases, four or six applications of the scissors may be necessary; the operation is painful, but is soon accomplished; as the wounds heal, contraction takes place, the aperture of the anus is diminished and braced up, and the prolapsus no longer occurs.

It is important to bear in mind that in very severe cases, not only is it necessary to remove the relaxed integument, but portions of the mucous membrane which, in instances of long standing, has become converted into a tissue more like leather than anything else, must also be taken away; if this step be not resorted to, a disappointment will ensue, as regards a complete remedy of the prolapsus. Hence the surgeon must think of the possibility of somewhat severe hæmorrhage, which will occasionally occur after a portion of the mucous membrane, however small, has been snipped away. I have seen it occur to a very great extent, and when it was least expected.

If hæmorrhage to a large extent does occur after a surgical operation on the rectum, the patient will in a few hours complain of tenesmus, and express a desire to go to the closet; he will then evacuate a large quantity of blood, and become faint. In such a case it will be necessary to clear away any coagula which may be in the gut, to elevate the pelvis, and introduce some ice into the bowel. Should this not stop the bleeding, a careful examination should be made with a speculum, if necessary, and the bleeding orifice be looked for, and tied. Sometimes it will be difficult or almost impossible to effect this, and then the rectum must be carefully plugged by portions of sponge or lint, to which a thread should be tied, in order that the compress may be more readily withdrawn when the bleeding has ceased.

It may here be stated that the risk of severe hæmorrhage, after the mucous membrane has been excised, may be in a great measure obviated by the surgeon taking care to introduce through the edges of each incision one or more fine sutures before the patient is left.

Another mode of curing prolapsus consists in the application of the ligature to portions of the prolapsed membrane. This plan is most especially adapted to those cases where there is great laxity of the mucous membrane, and the surrounding integument is not much involved; also to those cases, very numerous, where the prolapsus is associated with one or more hæmorrhoidal tumours. This operation was originally proposed for prolapsus by the late Mr. Copland, who found it to answer his expectations most admirably. It is easily done, by pinching up with a pair of forceps small portions of the diseased membrane, applying around each a tight thread, cutting off the extremities, and returning the parts within the sphincter. If there are distinct hæmorrhoidal tumours to deal with, the operation as undertaken for them, and described in another place, must be performed. As the prolapsus is in a great measure the result of the hæmorrhoids, the cure of the latter will be followed with the disappearance of the former.

CASE XIX.—The following is an instance of the cure of old prolapsus by ligature.

An officer in the army, aged forty-two, was sent to me, November, 1859, by Dr. Armstrong, of Blackrock. He had almost entirely lost the use of his bladder, being compelled to use the catheter three times a day; in addition to this great misfortune, he had a falling of the rectum, which had troubled him for twelve years, and which was increasing. The bowel protruded each time he went to the closet, necessitating its return by the hand of the patient, and sometimes this occurrence took place when he walked about; and there was a continual muco-purulent discharge which much annoyed him.

On examination, after an injection, I found that there was a portion of membrane, of considerable size, prolapsed on each side of the anus, that on the right being larger. The extremity of the prolapsed membrane, on either side, was indurated; whilst the upper portions were florid, and unchanged in appearance and texture. In addition, there were two or three small hæmorrhoidal excrescences, about the size of peas, just within the verge of the anus, and the integument was thickened and pendulous.

I gave this patient the option of either mode of treatment—by nitric acid or ligature—telling him, however, that in such a case there was much more certainty as to the effects of the latter than the former. He therefore assented to submit to the ligature, and on November 19th, having first emptied his bowels well by a large injection, and having got the part well protruded, I transfixed each of the prolapsed portions of mucous membrane with a needle carrying a double ligature, and tying the threads tightly, returned the bowel. I then snipped away with the scissors a greater portion of the pendulous flaps of integument. A dose of chalk and laudanum was given at night.

This patient did not suffer anything beyond a little distension of the belly. On the morning of the sixth day his bowels were well cleared, for the first time after the operation, by a dose of calomel, followed by castor-oil, the ligatures came away, and on the ninth day he was enabled to go out and dine at his club. His bowels acted naturally, without any prolapsus occurring.

There can be no particular objection to the employment of the ligature in persons not advanced in life, whose internal organs are sound, and whose constitutions have not been damaged by excesses, or by a long life in tropical climates. It appears to me, however, that when persons of the age of seventy and upwards are suffering from prolapsus, some other means of treatment less severe should be adopted. It may, however, happen that the surgeon is compelled, as it were, to adopt this operation in a case where the age and habit of the patient would otherwise preclude it. The prolapsed portion of bowel may have become irreducible, and those changes which prelude mortification of the parts may have set in, and be producing such symptoms as to induce the surgeon to hasten the process which nature has commenced. In the following instance, I applied the ligature where, under ordinary circumstances, there would have been grave objections to this proceeding.

CASE XX.—I was requested by Dr. Wildbore, February 26th, 1860, to see a lady, aged seventy, a large, stout woman, suffering from chronic bronchitis. On the day previous, a prolapsus of the rectum, from which she had suffered for many years, but which had been reducible, could not be got back; considerable pain and constitutional disturbance ensued. On examination, we found a considerable tumour, consisting mainly of the mucous membrane of the rectum, prolapsed and irreducible. One portion of the tumour, nearly as large as an egg, was in a semisloughy condition, and the patient was suffering severely both locally and constitutionally. It was useless to make any attempt to reduce the tumour in the state it was in, so we prescribed frequent poultices made of linseed meal and laudanum, and ordered opium internally.

On the following day we found that this treatment had had the effect of relieving the patient's sufferings, and subduing the local mischief. The sloughing process was, however, slowly going on, and it was thought most advisable to hasten this by ligaturing the whole mass; we determined, however, to wait another twenty-four hours, in order that the inflammation might be further subdued.

28th.—The ordinary operation by the ligature was performed this day, and the old lady was progressing favorably until the fourth day, when a copious hæmorrhage occurred from the parts operated upon, which lowered her very much, and increased her bronchitis. On examination it was ascertained that a slough had formed at the posterior border of the anus to the depth of three quarters of an inch, and had implicated one of the hæmorrhoidal arteries. I plugged this cavity most carefully with lint soaked in whisky, and as the old lady had been much prostrated by the bleeding, we prescribed wine and ammonia freely.

This case gave us some anxiety, especially as a second hæmorrhage occurred two days afterwards, but it was not so free, and did not return. The ligature separated on the eighth day, and the sloughing process had stopped; from this date the patient slowly but gradually rallied, and made an excellent recovery.

Now, in a case of this kind, where the patient was so old, and whose condition was so unfavorable for any surgical operation, it would, under any circumstances, be highly imprudent to apply the ligature; but as the prolapsed bowel had become irreducible, and a process which was more severe than that which the surgeon would adopt had set in, it was deemed most proper to hasten the separation of the prolapsed bowel by artificial means, for it was impossible to tell how long the natural process of sloughing would last, and whether the constitutional powers of the patient would bear up against it, whilst we knew, that after the application of the ligature, the separation of the diseased parts would be effected at the furthest in a few days, and there would be a less call upon the already-enfeebled powers of life. The nature of the bleeding here was somewhat curious, and it was due to the circumstance that the patient, who was very fat and heavy, lay continually on her back, and the pressure exerted just above the anus was the cause of the sloughing and subsequent hæmorrhage. We are taught a lesson by this case, viz., not to allow a patient under similar conditions to lie upon the back in one position.

In either of the operations just described, however, there is a certain amount of danger, and they compel a close confinement to bed and to the house for a week or two, and, therefore, if there is any other agent by which the prolapsus may be remedied, without producing either the danger to life or the confinement to bed, it should be adopted. The *strong nitric acid* which, locally applied to some forms of hæmorrhoids, is found to act so well, has lately been used by the author of this work in some severe and long-standing cases of prolapsus, with considerable success. It is, however, only in certain forms of the affection that the remedy will act with beneficial effects. In the cases of prolapsus of large size and of very long standing, where the mucous membrane has become very much thickened and changed in its structure and appearance, the acid will do little or no good; but in those cases of simple prolapsus of the bowel, where there are one or more large folds of mucous membrane continually down, and where the tissue is extremely vascular, presenting the appearance of smooth velvet, or is perhaps superficially ulcerated, and readily bleeds, the strong nitric acid, applied carefully to the whole or the greater portion of the diseased membrane will act like a charm. It should be used in the same manner, and with the same precautions, as when employed in instances of hæmorrhoids. If the entire surface of the prolapsed membrane be touched with it, one application alone will suffice to get rid of the disease; but it is better to apply the acid to a part only, and thus two or three operations may be necessary. This remedy, when carefully used, generally causes less pain than when it is applied to hæmorrhoids, for the mucous membrane, after having been long prolapsed, becomes much less sensitive than it usually is.

The following are instances where the nitric acid was attended with remarkable success:

CASE XXL—A man, aged seventy, applied at the Westminster General Dispensary, August 24th, 1854. He presented the aspect of severe suffering. He had been a sufferer from prolapsus of the rectum for a period of twenty years, and latterly the protrusion had increased so much, that he was unable to return it after the bowels had been moved. There was constant protrusion, and he suffered much from pain. But the chief source of his misery was the circumstance of his having almost entirely lost control over the sphincter, so that the contents of the bowels escaped involuntarily.

On examination I discovered that there was a considerable swelling at the anus, consisting externally of loose and thickened integument, and within this, of the mucous membrane of the rectum; highly vascular and relaxed, but not changed much as regards its actual character.

I cleansed the parts well with dry lint, and applied the strong nitric acid to the whole of the protruded membrane, smeared the part abundantly with oil, and returned it within the sphincter. The patient suffered considerably, but it was mainly from my efforts to return the prolapsed intestine.

I saw this patient on the 30th. He had had one evacuation, and stated he had more control over the sphincter. On examination, I found the protrusion much less; the mucous membrane was corrugated and hardened. I therefore applied the acid again.

At the patient's next visit to the dispensary in a few days, I was absent, but he saw the house-surgeon, and informed him that he was better than he had been for twenty years. This gentleman applied the acid a third time.

October 9th.—This man came to-day. His countenance indicated a mind at ease, and renovated health. He informed me that he was well, and on examination I could not discover a trace of the protrusion.

CASE XXII.—Colonel B—, aged seventy-three (sent by Mr. Peter Hood), applied to me, July 23rd, 1859. He informed me that, so long ago as thirty years, he suffered from hæmorrhoids and prolapsus, and applied to the late Mr. Copeland, who operated on him by the ligature and scissors with very good effect. He did not again suffer until the last three years, when the disease reappeared. He has had a descent of the bowels generally when at the closet, and latterly when he stands or walks about. On examination I found a large prolapsus of the mucous membrane on the right side, and on the left side was one distinct hæmorrhoidal tumour of considerable size. The mucous membrane, at the upper portion of the prolapsus, was highly vascular, and unaltered in its character, whilst a portion of it at the inferior extremity, was thickened, and transformed almost into integument.

I applied the acid carefully to the upper portion of the prolapsed membrane; the patient did not feel the application.

25th.—No pain or irritation followed this operation. I applied the acid again.

27th.—No ill effects; the patient now finds the bowel come down less when at the closet, and it does not protrude at all when he walks about. On examination I could not see any protrusion, I therefore introduced the speculum, and applied the acid again.

29th.—He now suffers nothing from the protrusion, which scarcely comes down at all, even at the closet. I introduced the speculum, and applied the acid for the fourth and last time.

This gentleman wrote to me from abroad some little time after, to thank me for my most successful treatment of his case.

This gentleman called on me some months afterwards. I found there was a slight protrusion of the mucous membrane, to which I applied the nitric acid again.

CASE XXIII.—The Rev. Mr. C—, aged fifty, consulted me November 24th. He informed me that he had suffered from disease about the rectum for many years. Eight years previously he had undergone the operation of the ligature, for what he termed piles, at the hands of a surgeon in a provincial town. After recovery from this operation, he experienced but slight relief, and he continued to suffer more or less from relaxation and protrusion of the bowel. Since this period he placed himself under the care of one or two surgeons of large experience, and, in addition, placed himself in a hydropathic establishment, but he obtained no benefit.

On examination, after he had been seated over hot water, I found that there was a large prolapsus of the entire circumference of the mucous membrane of the rectum, dark and congested, but smooth, and not altered in its essential character, there being no induration whatever. There was a considerable quantity of relaxed and thickened skin around the margin of the anus. The sphincter was very much relaxed. I have seldom noticed a case where there was more relaxation. The general health of this gentleman was not strong. He complained of a great weakness in his legs at times, and he walked as though he was semi-paralysed. He informed me that he also suffered much more from the protrusion of the rectum at one time than another, more especially when he had any particular mental work or annoyance. He also informed me, that at times he was hardly conscious of the contents of the rectum passing.

Although the ligature had been applied here, and had been followed by the return or persistence of the prolapsus, I strongly recommended that the patient should submit to it again, and that the relaxed skin around the anus should be removed. I was induced to give this advice, because there was so much relaxation of the parts, and I suspect that in the former operation the very important step of removing the relaxed folds of skin had been neglected. The patient however was averse to this proceeding, and asked if any hopes could be held out of the nitric acid doing good. He was informed that relief could be certainly effected, perhaps complete.

On the 25th, after the bowel had been well got down, I applied the nitric acid carefully to one portion of the prolapsed membrane. This application he did not feel; he was desired to lie quiet on the sofa for an hour or two.

28th.—He did not feel any pain from the acid, but there was some little difficulty in micturition, and there has been some smartish bleeding from the rectum, when at the closet; but already he has noticed a diminution of the prolapsus. On examination I found the portion of mucous membrane upon which the acid had been applied superficially ulcerated, and the volume of the gut decidedly less.

30th.—There has not been any protrusion since—by sitting over hot water, however, the patient was able to protrude the bowel, and I carefully applied the nitric acid to a part of the mucous membrane which had not been previously touched.

December 2nd.—No pain followed this application; he has not had any protrusion, and it is with great difficulty that any of the bowel is forced down, and then it returns immediately. I applied the acid to a small portion of the mucous membrane. On the following day I removed the relaxed skin around the anus with scissors.

8th.—He visited me to-day, stating that he has not had any prolapsus whatever; and on examination I found no protrusion of the bowel, and the wounds made by the scissors cicatrizing healthily. This gentleman expressed himself as much satisfied. I enjoined him to be particular about the action of his bowels, ordering him to take occasionally two drachms of the mixed confection of black pepper and senna. I also advised him to throw up the rectum four ounces of the sulphate of iron lotion two or three times a week, and to continue it for some period.

This case particularly shows the good results which ensue from the application of the nitric acid in a very severe form of prolapsus, where the mucous membrane has not become indurated or otherwise much altered in its texture. If the tissue had been thickened or infiltrated with deposit of lymph, as is so frequently the case in old prolapsus, there would not have been any appreciable benefit; in fact, I should not have tried the acid, knowing from experience its uselessness in such a condition. When, however, the mucous membrane is soft and velvety—however large be the prolapsus—the acid will bring about a cure or very great relief. Neither of these results, however, will be satisfactory unless the redundant skin around the margin of the anus be removed.

CASE XXIV.—Mr. H—, aged thirty-eight, consulted me December 10th. He informed me that he suffered for several years from hæmorrhage from the rectum. This had ceased for more than a year; since this time, however, he has been annoyed with prolapse of the bowel. It always descended when he was at the closet; and, of late, the gut remained down for a considerable time, varying from half an hour to three hours; when, by the aid of a sponge and cold water, it returned; during this period the uneasiness and suffering were great, but after the prolapse was put back all the symptoms disappeared. He has, on one or two occasions, been laid up with an acute attack of the disease, which has confined him to bed for some weeks. Various remedies have been tried, but none have been of any service to him.

On examination, I found that there presented at the anus, without any expulsive effort, on either side a flap of dark, smooth, velvety mucous membrane, which was, however, so thickly covered with a dark mucous discharge that at first I thought the disease was a distinct hæmorrhoidal tumour. On carefully cleansing the parts, the swelling was found to consist of two folds of membrane, surrounded by a large quantity of loose and indurated integument. The patient informed me that the discharge was very abundant, and annoyed him exceedingly.

11th.—Having this morning well cleared the rectum out by an enema, and brought all the prolapsed membrane down,

I applied the nitric acid, and returned it. The patient did not feel the application of the remedy.

13th.—He has had no pain, and the discharge is much less. There is no prolapse visible. I therefore employed the speculum, and touched a small portion of the mucous membrane with the acid.

15th.—This patient walked about a great deal yesterday, took several glasses of spirit-and-water, and had an aperient draught in the evening, which has acted powerfully this morning; and, on examination, there is a small portion of mucous membrane prolapsed, contrary to my expectation. I therefore applied the acid again; and, having done this, and sent him home to bed, I clipped away the greater portion of the thickened skin around the anus.

17th.—He walked to my house this morning, and on examination no prolapse is visible.

This gentleman wrote to me in a week, from the country, to say that his bowels now "acted naturally, without pain, bleeding, or protrusion." I enjoined him to be careful about keeping his bowels regular, and recommended him to use the sulphate of iron injection occasionally at night time. I saw this gentleman in January, 1862. He informed me he was perfectly well.

Since the publication of the last edition of this work, I have met with a considerable number of old-standing and severe cases of prolapsus of the rectum, where, either from the existence of some organic disease, or from advanced age, the operation by the ligature was not admissible, and yet, from the extent and nature of the disorder, it could not be remedied by the application of nitric acid alone. Under such circumstances I have adopted what may be considered a combined method of treatment, consisting in the employment of nitric acid, and in the removal of folds of relaxed tissue from around the margin of the anus. I published at length some observations on this point, and some illustrative cases in the 'Medical Times and Gazette,' for September 14th, 1861.

It is mainly in those cases where there is considerable prolapsus in weak or old persons, associated with a very relaxed condition of the anal orifice, that I adopt this practice, which I can recommend with confidence. The nitric acid should be applied first, as often as may be needful, and when the prolapsed membrane has become reduced as much as possible by the action of this remedy, two, three, or more strips of the relaxed skin should be removed from the margin of the anus and at right angles to that orifice. The operation is affected by seizing the part to be removed by a hooked forceps in the left hand, whilst, with a pair of sharp scissors, curved on the flat, the raised tissue is rapidly removed. In cases where the anal orifice is much dilated, and the mucous membrane at the base of the prolapse has become much indurated, the points of the scissors may be dipped well down into the orifice, so as to remove a portion of this indurated membrane as well as the integument.

The result of this treatment is, that as cicatrization of the wounds proceeds, the anus becomes contracted and braced up, and when the mucous membrane has previously been well acted upon by the application of the nitric acid, nearly as good an effect has been produced as though the ligature had been used, and the inconveniences and dangers of the latter operation have been escaped, for although I look upon the ligature in healthy persons and in those not very advanced in life as an extremely safe and satisfactory proceeding, it must be admitted by all that where the contrary conditions obtain, it is not free from serious risks.

The following well illustrates the kind of case alluded to, and the beneficial effects of the treatment adopted.

CASE XXV.—Mr. B—, aged fifty-four, sent to me by Mr. Fereday, of Dudley, December 7th, 1860. He had been suffering for several years from hæmorrhage and prolapse of the rectum. The former symptom had gradually subsided, but during the last two years the bowel had been almost constantly protruded, and the pain attending the disease had been very great. On examining him after the parts had been well brought down by an injection, I found a large tumour composed externally of a quantity of relaxed and thickened integument, and within that, of two lateral flaps of thickened granular and highly vascular mucous membrane. There were no hæmorrhoidal tumours. The anal orifice was extremely capacious, and the most distressing symptom this patient complained of was the inability to control his evacuations.

In other respects this gentleman was in a very shaky condition, suffering from great difficulty of breathing and irregular action of the heart. He had also had considerable enlargement of the liver and œdema of the legs, and was altogether about as unfavorable a subject as could be desired for undergoing any surgical operation, and yet his local miseries were so great as to necessitate some measure for his relief.

It would have been most imprudent to adopt the ligature in such a case, even had the patient consented to it, and therefore I determined to put in force the combined method of treatment just described, holding out the hope that the patient would be relieved of all the most distressing symptoms at least, and perhaps cured. Accordingly, on the same evening, I began the treatment by applying the nitric acid to the mucous membrane, and repeated the same two days afterwards.

13th.—The nitric acid having reduced the prolapsus very much, I this day removed from around the margin of the anus four folds of relaxed integument, having previously benumbed the part with ice and salt.

16th.—The bowels have been kept quiet until to-day,

when they were acted upon by castor oil, only a slight protrusion occurring.

19th.—The wounds made by the scissors have nearly healed, so I made a further application of the nitric acid to a portion of mucous membrane which could be protruded. This was repeated again on the 22nd and 26th. On the last occasion, I found that what protrusion remained was returned by the least pressure, and that the sphincter contracted in a much more healthy manner. He is to return home in a day or two. I recommended him to pass a bougie every day after his bowels have been opened, and to use the sulphate of iron lotion.

This gentleman wrote to me in six weeks' time, to say that he had walked several times a distance of one or two miles without any return of the complaint, and was "quite a new creature." Six months afterwards he called upon me to say he was quite well.

Whilst speaking of the treatment of hæmorrhoidal tumours, I described a method of removing them, which consists of a combination of excision and nitric acid. I deferred the relation of any cases treated in this way until I was considering the subject of prolapsus, because the application of the remedy is just the same in the one affection as in the other, and is used in a precisely similar manner. I have already described the manner in which it is adopted, and the instruments which are used. I must, however, mention here that the clamp, as ordinarily made, has not seemed to me to be sufficiently adapted for the purpose intended. The edges are serrated, and do not meet so as to compress the base of the tumour with sufficient tightness. I have, therefore, re-

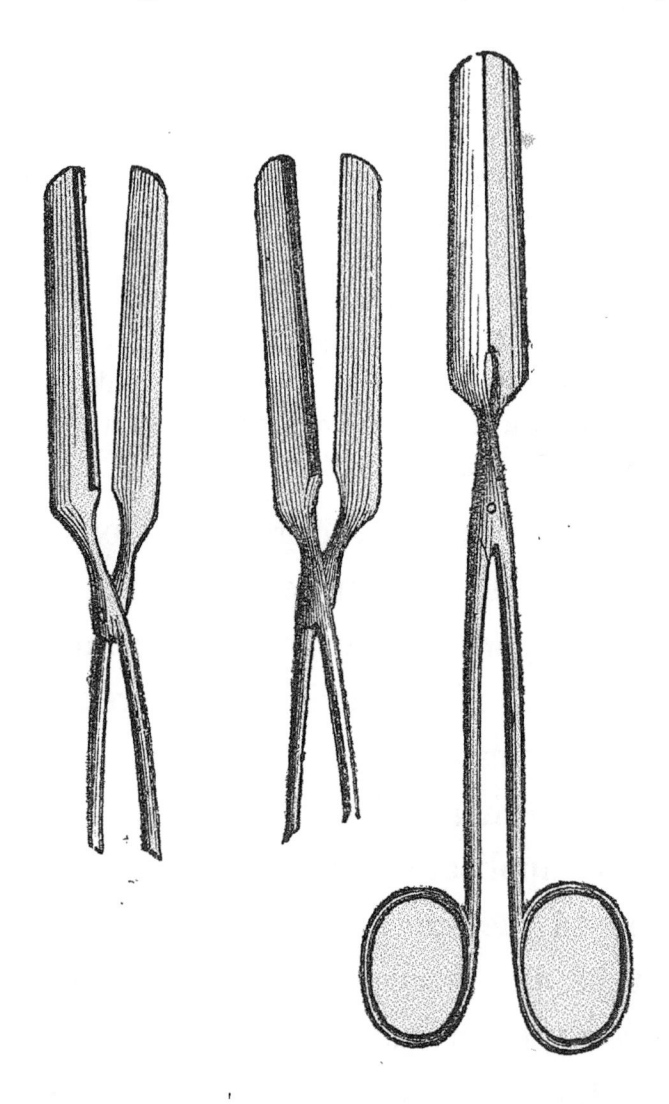

quested **Mr.** Matthews to construct these clamps in such a manner as to produce the most thorough compression upon the tissue which they hold in their grasp, and thus prevent the possibility of hæmorrhage. Mr. Matthews has effected this by grooving one of the blades of the instrument, so that when the two are brought together not the slightest interval exists between the raised surface on the one and the groove in the other.

If this operation be done with great care, there is very little pain attending it, the only suffering the patient complains of is when the part is first seized and compressed by the clamp. The subsequent stages of excising the prominent portion of the hæmorrhoid or prolapsus, and of applying the nitric acid, are of necessity painless, because the part exposed is deprived of all sensibility, in consequence of the powerful compression exercised by the clamp. It is necessary to keep the patient in bed or on the sofa for two days, otherwise considerable irritation and even inflammation might be produced.

My experience of this mode of treatment leads me to speak in very high terms of it; the results are as favorable as those obtained by the ligature, and there is certainly less suffering and less risk of unpleasant consequences. It may be looked upon as a proceeding perfectly free from danger; when executed in a cautious and proper manner, and when the hæmorrhoidal tumours are limited in size, or the prolapsed part does not involve a large portion of the bowel, it may be recommended to the patient with the greatest confidence.

I will now detail a few cases illustrating the value of this mode of treatment.

CASE XXVI.—A military officer, aged seventy, who had served in India for many years, consulted me in July last for hæmorrhoids and prolapsus. He had suffered many years, but it was only latterly that he had been seriously annoyed, in consequence of the protrusion occurring whenever he took exercise.

On examination, I found a large protrusion of mucous membrane on the right side, vascular and healthy, and on the left side was a large hæmorrhoidal tumour, nearly as big as a walnut, of a deep blue colour, and mainly consisting of venous tissue. I applied nitric acid on four different occasions to the prolapsed mucous membrane, after which it disappeared. I then proposed to my patient that the hæmorrhoidal tumour should be treated by the clamp and nitric acid, and, accordingly, I adopted this method, first seizing the base of the tumour, compressing it well, and, whilst my assistant held the clamp firmly, I removed the prominent portion of the mass, and touched the raw surface most thoroughly with the nitric acid, and having kept it exposed for a short time, returned it. The patient scarcely felt any pain; no bleeding ensued; he lay quiet for forty-eight hours, and quickly recovered. At the end of a fortnight the patient called on me, to say he had no protrusion at all. In January last, six months after the treatment, he called on me to say he was quite well, and had not been so comfortable for thirty years.

This case is particularly instructive, because it shows the value of nitric acid alone for one particular part of the disease—the prolapsus; whilst for the hæmorrhoidal tumour it would have been powerless alone, and nothing but the ligature would have been of any use in the absence of the treatment I adopted.

When several tumours instead of one require to be treated, the method in question, although resulting in equal success, requires much more care at the hand of the surgeon, and is not so simple. In the following case, one of the most recent treated by me in this manner, there were no less than four distinct tumours operated upon:

CASE XXVII.—A gentleman, aged fifty, consulted me in March last. He had suffered many years from hæmorrhage from the rectum and protrusion. He was also the subject of asthma, and was not a healthy man. On examination, I found a bunch of four hæmorrhoidal tumours protruding at the anus; they were of a bright scarlet colour, easily bleeding, and of the particular character for which nitric acid alone was well adapted; but the tumours were prominent, and had distinct pedicles, numerous applications of nitric acid would have been necessary. I did not recommend the ligature, because the patient was not a sound man; but I advised him to undergo the treatment by the clamp and nitric acid. Accordingly, on March 9th, in company with Mr. Swayne, of Erith, I performed the operation, by successively compressing each of the tumours with the clamp, removing them with sharp scissors, and then applying the acid. Scarcely any pain was felt; there was hardly any bleeding. The patient kept his bed for two days, and was able, in a little more than a week, to come to London to attend to his business. He called upon me within the fortnight, stating he had no prolapsus or hæmorrhage, and, in a few days more, was quite well.

Although this method of treatment is perhaps better adapted for cases of hæmorrhoids where the tumours are distinct and defined, it is almost equally useful in instances of prolapsus of the rectum, where a resort to the nitric acid alone will not be followed by satisfactory results. I have before stated that I have been disappointed with the action of nitric acid in some cases where it was tried with care, and the failure has for the most part occurred when the agent has been applied in cases of pure prolapsus. Considerable benefit has been produced at first, but subsequently the symptoms have returned, and the patients have been obliged to submit to the ligature, either at my own hands or at those of others, and thus discredit has been thrown upon a most useful remedy. I will, however, candidly admit that the good effects which have been produced in well-selected cases led me to try it in instances where I should not now think of using it. When, then, these doubtful cases come before me, and the patient will not submit to the ligature, or this proceeding is not admissible, I employ the method now under notice. The case I now relate illustrates its value well.

CASE XXVIII.—A gentleman, aged fifty, long resident in India, consulted me, March 6th. He was in feeble health, and had been troubled for some years from prolapsus of the rectum, which occurred each time he visited the closet, and annoyed him a good deal.

On examination, I found a considerable prolapse of the mucous membrane on the right side, very vascular, but smooth, and not indurated. This was surrounded by a thick belt of membrane consisting of the muco-cutaneous lining at the edge of the sphincter. This patient was indisposed to undergo the operation of the ligature, and I therefore recommended him to be treated by the clamp and nitric acid. Accordingly, on March 7th, having first seized and well compressed the base of the protruded membrane with the clamp, I removed the free portion with sharp scissors; the incised surface, which was rather extensive, was then carefully wiped and exposed for some minutes, and the nitric acid was freely applied. I then snipped off the most redundant portions of the œdematous ring at the verge of the anus. There was very little suffering at the time of the operation.

This gentleman experienced a gnawing sensation for some hours after the operation, but no other unpleasant symptoms. He kept his bed for two days; the first action of the bowels, on the fourth day, was accompanied by smarting. On the sixth day he was enabled to dine at his club, and ten days after the operation he left London. A fortnight afterwards he wrote to me saying that he had caught cold, had experienced a most violent attack of diarrhœa, which, to use his own words, "tested the efficacy of my treatment well;" but it had produced no return of the old symptoms, nor, in fact, any local suffering whatever.

It must be admitted by every surgeon who has had much practical experience, that there is no class of diseases of a painful and distressing character which admit of relief and cure so readily as those affecting the rectum; and yet it is curious to witness the immense amount of annoyance and suffering which well-educated and informed persons have undergone for many years of their life, from a conviction that the science of surgery either cannot relieve them of their malady, or that the dangers attending the necessary treatment are essentially great. Thus it is that we not unfrequently meet with instances of prolapsus of the rectum, which have attained an immense size, and which have existed for a long series of years. In the majority of these cases the patients are far gone in years, and indeed are so accustomed to the existence of the prolapse, that comparatively little distress is produced. It will however happen now and then that some relief must be afforded in such cases, and any operation is out of the question. The protrusion, in fact, is of very large size, and the tissues are exceedingly indurated, and the anal orifice is relaxed and capacious; the general health also is feeble. The only remedies which can be of service are, a careful attention to the bowels, and the employment of well-made pessaries. They often fail in the purpose of keeping the parts in their proper situation, but at the same time I have known some old people obtain the greatest comfort from them.

THE PAINFUL ULCER OF THE RECTUM.

That peculiar form of ulceration met with at the extremity of the rectum, and usually known by the name of Fissure of the Anus, or Irritable Ulcer of the Rectum, is worthy of special attention, insomuch as it is not uncommonly associated with hæmorrhoidal disease, is frequently mistaken for that or other morbid affection, and is productive of perhaps more suffering than any other disorder of so local and limited a nature.

The pathology of this affection is somewhat obscure. It is probable that the disease is produced in the following manner:—The patient suffers more or less from habitual constipation, and during the straining efforts which take place, a slight rent of the mucous membrane occurs, and, in consequence of the periodical movements of the lower part of the bowel and the passage of hardened fæces, the breach of surface becomes more extensive, and is prevented from healing, and that which at first is only a linear fissure, becomes a decided ulcer. The formation of such an ulcer is, moreover, favoured by the peculiar constitution of the bowel, which, at its lower extremity, presents several sinuses or pouches, in which fæcal matter or other foreign bodies are liable to be entangled. It is not uncommonly noticed, also, that one or more hæmorrhoidal excrescences are seen at the verge of the anus in connection with the painful ulcer, and it is very probable that the disease in question is originally produced by the mere mechanical impediment of fæcal and other matters at the base of these tumours, which, begetting irritation and local inflammation, lead on to the formation of small circumscribed spots of ulceration. The view that constipation is the most favorable cause of the painful ulcer derives strength from the circumstance that the affection is met with most frequently in women, who generally suffer from constipation more than persons of the opposite sex.

The symptoms complained of by those who labour under this affection are well marked and peculiar, so much so that it is surprising to meet with cases where the malady has not been suspected, much less discovered by the medical attendant. In many cases the patient complains of more or less acute pain during the time that the contents of the rectum are being evacuated; this increases and becomes aggravated after the action of the bowels, and lasts for a period of one or more hours, after which it subsides. In other instances the pain is not experienced during the time of defæcation, but after an interval varying from ten minutes to an hour the pain comes on, and is increased until it is described as actual torture. In one case which I recently saw, the suffering was so acute a short time after the action of the bowels, that the patient writhed in torture, and required large doses of opium to relieve him. When these sufferings have been endured for several hours, a complete subsidence ensues, and there is a freedom from pain until the next call to the closet, when a similar condition of suffering is produced. At first the general health is not much affected, but after the disease has lasted for a period of some months, the constitution begins to suffer unmistakeably. The patient becomes pale, sallow, and listless; complains of pains in the loins and down the thighs, and is very frequently reduced to a great extent of debility. In women the symptoms are so like those dependent upon uterine disease, that not unfrequently the real disorder has been overlooked, and repeated local applications have been made to the womb, whilst in reality the rectum has been the offending part.

When the disorder has lasted for some length of time, there is a slight discharge of purulent fluid streaked with blood, but in some instances the attention of the patient is not directed to this symptom.

In one well-marked case which I saw some little time since, the only thing the patient complained of was a considerable irritation of the anus; there was not any pain. On examination I discovered a small ulcer at the verge of the anus, which had evidently existed for a long period.

When a patient presents with the symptoms of this ulcer, the most careful examination should be instituted, for the real nature of the affection, especially in certain instances, may be readily overlooked. He should be made to kneel down, or, if a female, to lie down on the side, with the buttocks well exposed to a good light; the surgeon should then gently and carefully expose the anal orifice, and desire the patient to make a straining effort. If the disease exist, its anal extremity will come into view, and will look exactly like a simple fissure or rent. If, however, the patient further protrudes the parts, and some little force is employed in separating the sides of the anus with the thumbs, the edges of the fissure will diverge, and its true character will be observed. Not unfrequently a small tumour or hæmorrhoidal excresence will be found at the verge of the anus; and on well exposing this, the fissure or ulcer will be seen at its base, hid, as it were, behind it. In fact, the existence of this small tumour is a pretty correct indication of the presence of the ulcer.

The situation, form, and appearance of the ulcer differs. Thus, in one instance, the discase may be so located as to be almost entirely without the verge of the anus, implicating the sphincter but slightly, and be readily brought into view. In another case it may be seated quite across the fibres of the sphincter muscle, and then only a portion of the ulcerated surface can be brought into view. The shape of the ulcer varies—it is round, oval, or triangular, generally measuring from the eighth of an inch to half an inch in length. Its surface presents in one case the appearance of a bright red colour, in another a grayish colour. When the disease is recent, the edges are level with the ulcer; if, however, it has existed for any length of time, the borders are raised and indurated.

Sometimes there are two ulcers, or rather one ulcer is separated into two portions by a process of integument. Thus, in one instance recently under my care, there were found to be two small hæmorrhoidal excrescences at the verge of the anus, situated about half an inch apart. On separating the sides of the anus, a large ulceration of a triangular form was seen, its base being bounded by the two tumours, and its apex running into the bowel, and through the centre ran a raised process of integument, which almost completely produced the formation of two ulcers.

When the ulcer or fissure is situated within the external sphincter muscle, or when there is much contraction and spasm of the part, it is difficult to get a view of it, or only a portion of the abraded surface can be seen. Most valuable information may in this case be obtained by the use of the finger, introduced carefully into the bowel, when the peculiar rough sensation is imparted to it, which can hardly be described, but which cannot well be mistaken. In most cases, too, when the finger of the surgeon is introduced, the patient experiences most acute pain, which fact greatly assists the diagnosis.

Every now and then a patient will complain of the well-marked symptoms of this disorder, and yet, on examination, nothing can be seen or even felt beyond, perhaps, a slight roughness at some particular spot of mucous membrane well within the sphincter. Even an examination by the speculum may fail to detect any decided ulceration. These cases are rare; but one occurred to me only the other day. The symptoms were well marked, and yet I could detect nothing like ulceration even with the speculum; but, on introducing the finger, a very slight roughness was observed at one spot, and the contact of the finger produced violent pain. This gentleman had previously consulted two well-known surgeons, one of whom had affirmed that an ulcer existed. The other gave the contrary opinion.

In by far the majority of cases the painful ulcer is met with at the posterior verge of the anus, nearly or quite in the median line.

I think, I may state, from my own experience, that in nine-tenths of the cases the ulcer has been found thus situated. Now and then, but rarely, it is met with in the front and in the middle, and occasionally it is seen on one side.

Although the painful ulcer of the rectum is productive of the utmost amount of suffering, it may be remedied more easily, perhaps, than any other severe disorder. In those cases where the ulcer is seated so low down as to be within the view of the surgeon, the careful application of the solid nitrate of silver from time to time will bring about a cure. Several applications may be necessary, and no other remedial measure will be required; but, should this not succeed, an ointment made of the cinereous oxide of mercury, in the proportion of half a drachm of the mineral to one ounce of lard, should be used. In other instances the daily introduction of a full-sized bougie made of wax or of yellow soap will be followed by the best results. During the time that these agents are employed, great care should be taken to produce a proper action of the bowels, and a healthy state of the secretions by small doses of calomel and rhubarb.

I have succeeded, in some severe cases, in bringing about a cure by a careful application of such means as I have just mentioned. The following is a good illustration of the beneficial effect of the nitrate of silver in a case where more severe means could not be adopted.

CASE XXVIII.—Mr. B—, aged forty-nine, suffering from diabetes, called on me in January. He had been under the care of a gentleman who had had his attention more particularly directed to the state of his general health, and had not ascertained the existence of any disease in the rectum, although the patient had complained of pain and uneasiness there. He had been suffering for more than two years from pain after the action of the bowels, and on examination, I discovered an ulcer situated on the sphincter, about half an inch in length and the eighth of an inch in breadth; its edges presented the appearance of a chronic ulcer of the leg, being raised, thick, and indurated. Much suffering and annoyance was caused by the existence of this affection, but as the general health was so reduced by the diabetes, it was considered imprudent to perform any operation; therefore, I carefully applied the solid nitrate of silver to the ulcer, and repeated it twice weekly for five weeks with a gradual improvement, until the end of this period, when the ulceration had quite healed. During this period I desired the patient to pay great attention to the state of the bowels, and to refrain from any stimulating diet.

I believe that many cases of the painful ulcer may be treated satisfactorily in this way, especially when the disease is so situated as to be brought readily into view, but when such is not the case, and when there is associated with it — as frequently occurs — a spasmodic contraction of the sphincter ani, a surgical operation is required. It is, however, one of a simple character, and most certainly resulting in success, if properly performed. The French surgeon, Boyer, to whom we are indebted for the correct treatment of this disease by operation, acted upon that sound principle which is now so much recognised in the adoption of surgical means, and which consists in keeping parts diseased or injured, and liable to be injuriously affected by motion, in a state of perfect quiescence. He practised the division of the sphincter muscle, and the painful ulcer, being no longer affected by muscular movement, was found to heal. The operation in his hands was, however, a somewhat severe business, as a large wound was made; but now, thanks to the suggestion of the late Mr. Copeland, surgeons, whilst recognising the same principle as influenced Boyer, are content with making only a limited incision, so as to fairly cut through the ulcer, and only divide a portion of the fibres of the sphincter muscle. Some surgeons even suppose that it is not necessary to divide any of the fibres of the sphincter, and simply recommend an incision through the ulcer; but it must be borne in mind that a fair incision to the bottom of the ulcer will of necessity involve some portion of the sphincter. The rule I adopt and would recommend is, to carry the incision to such an extent as will produce a sensible dilation of the anal orifice. This is readily ascertained by introducing the finger after the operation. If the ulcer be fairly divided, and with it some of the fibres of the sphincter, the contraction of the lower part of the bowel will be much diminished when the finger is introduced, and this is a pretty certain indication that the necessary incision has been affected.

The operation is very simple. Whilst the patient is lying on the side the surgeon introduces his left fore-finger, well oiled, into the rectum, turning its bulb to the direction of the ulcer. He then introduces a narrow, straight probe-pointed bistoury, flat along the finger, until its point has reached beyond the extremity of the fissure, when it is turned round with the cutting edge against the sore; and as it is brought out, the necessary incision is made. If there be any hæmorrhoidal excrescences or flaps of skin coexistent with the ulcer, these should be removed with the scissors. A small strip of oiled lint may be introduced to keep the wound apart, but this is not necessary. I invariably pass up a suppository made of pil. saponis co., and extract of hyoscyamus, six grains of each, immediately after the operation. Of course the bowels should be well cleared out both by medicine and enema before the operation, as there is much less chance of any action occurring until a period of three or four days has elapsed. The good result of this proceeding will be seen when the bowels are first moved by medicine. The peculiar pain which was so distressing previously, and which lasted, perhaps, for half an hour or an hour, will be replaced by the smarting caused by the passage of fæcal matter over a raw surface, and which subsides in a few minutes. On the second occasion, perhaps, even this will not be felt, and, in the majority of cases, the cure will be complete in a fortnight. Sometimes it will be necessary to dress the wound with some stimulating lotion, and to give some of the confection of black pepper, but, after a large experience, I have seldom found these remedies called for.

I will now give some examples of the cure of this disease by operation.

CASE XXIX.—Mr. P—, aged forty-four, sent for me, February 12th, 1860. He had been suffering from some painful affection of the rectum for some time, and when I saw him he was confined to his bed, and his countenance betokened great distress. His symptoms were well marked and indicative of the disease in question, but there was this peculiarity about them—the pain which he experienced did not come on until about one hour after the bowels had been moved, when it attacked him with great severity, and lasted for a period varying from six to eight hours, after which he was perfectly free from suffering until after the next evacuation. He had been treated, as I find many such cases are, for external piles, but, of course, he had not experienced any relief.

On examination, I found that he had a hæmorrhoidal state of the lower part of the rectum, but feeling satisfied that this would not account for the peculiar symptoms, I caused the patient to protrude the parts as much as possible, and I then detected an ulcer at the posterior verge of the anus. Its surface was florid, and easily bled; the edges were thick and indurated. The introduction of the finger gave excessive pain.

February 14th.—I this day fairly divided the ulcer, the incision involving some of the fibres of the sphincter.

19th.—His bowels were kept locked up by opium until yesterday, when they were moved by castor oil without pain. The wound is looking well, and discharging freely.

27th.—This gentleman called on me to-day, looking vastly altered for the better. He had lost the anxious cast of countenance, and has informed me that he had entirely got rid of his painful sensations when the bowels were moved.

This disease is liable to be overlooked, more especially in females, as the symptoms in them are more severe and complex, and not unfrequently referred to the uterus, or, if it be accompanied with hæmorrhoids or prolapsus, is treated for either of these affections.

In the following case the nature of the disorder was entirely overlooked, and produced most distressing symptoms.

CASE XXX.—I was requested to see, in September, 1859, a single lady, aged twenty-five, who had been confined to her bed for some time with an affection of the rectum. She had been troubled with prolapsus for two years, and, consequently, the present symptoms were referred to this disorder. Various kinds of treatment, including leeches, had been used in vain. She had severe pain when the bowels acted; this increased afterwards, and became agonising, lasting for hours, when it subsided. The general health was much pulled down.

On examination, a single hæmorrhoidal excrescence was seen at the posterior verge of the anus, and concealed by this was a fissure, which, when the borders of the orifice were drawn aside, was found to be an ulcer of the bowel, with a smooth, florid surface and raised edges. On introducing the finger great agony was caused, and the peculiar rough feeling was imparted to the touch.

On the next day I fairly divided the ulcer, together with some fibres of the sphincter, after the patient had been placed under chloroform. Four days afterwards I visited her, and found the most marked change in her appearance. She expressed herself as having had complete relief from the operation, and a fortnight subsequently I saw her medical attendant, who informed me she had regained her health and strength.

In the following case the disease was supposed to be referred to the uterus and one of the sequelæ of parturition, and the medical gentleman who attended the lady in her confinement was unjustly blamed for having been the cause of the symptoms.

CASE XXXI.—I was requested by a physician in London, in November last, to see a married lady, aged twenty-five, who had been suffering much since her confinement, three months previously, from painful symptoms about the lower part of the pelvis. As they were not well defined, it was supposed that they depended upon some injury in the labour. I ascertained that there was almost constant pain about the rectum, both before and after the action of the bowels, and that this was much aggravated by any movement. The signs were not clearly indicative of an ulcer of the bowel, but on instituting an examination, I discovered a small fissure just within the verge of the anus, and so situated that on the patient protruding the parts its whole extent could be well seen. As it was very slight, I endeavoured to heal it with nitrate of silver, but after two or three applications no benefit accrued. Accordingly, on the 21st, I divided the ulcer fairly. On visiting her two days subsequently, the bowels had been opened without pain. This relief continued, the wound put on a healing appearance, and in a few days she got quite well.

I have in my own practice met with more cases of painful ulcer of the rectum in women than in men, and certainly the suffering is much more marked in them than in the opposite sex. Why it is so I cannot explain, any more than I can the undoubted fact that women suffer much more from the effects of hæmorrhoids, and from the surgical treatment which is adopted. I have, however, occasionally seen the most serious sufferings produced by the ulcer of the rectum in men, and the most severe of the kind was one I recently had under my care in King's College Hospital.

CASE XXXII.—A labouring man, aged fifty, was admitted into the Hospital in September. He had been suffering for several months with the most aggravated symptoms of ulcer of the rectum, consisting in severe pain at the time the bowels were relieved, continuing afterwards for an hour and more, and recurring daily. There was a discharge of blood and pus from the bowel. Nothing was visible externally, but on introducing the finger an ulcer as large as a sixpence was found on the posterior surface of the rectum, implicating the external sphincter, but extending within it. The introduction of the finger produced actual torture. I tried various measures to produce relief in this case, such as the use of suppositories, the cinereous oxide of mercury ointment, and the passing of bougies, but they were absolutely powerless. Accordingly, on the 14th, I divided the ulcer very freely, cutting through a considerable portion of the fibres of the sphincter. The relief, as is usual, was speedy. On the first action of the bowels there was scarcely any pain; the wound healed up well, and the man left in about a fortnight, and he subsequently presented himself to me to tell me he was quite well.

Now and then cases are met with where there are one or more cracks present in the radiating folds of skin at the margin of the anus, not involving the sphincter, and very superficial. I have seen much annoyance caused by them, and sometimes they are difficult to heal. The most appropriate treatment is the prevention of constipation, the ablution of the parts with soap and water, and the application of a strong solution of nitrate of silver by means of a brush. I have had occasion, in one or two obstinate cases, to make an incision through them, as in the ordinary painful ulcer.

Small ulcers are not unfrequently seen amongst our hospital out-patients, as the result of gonorrhœal and venereal matters coming into contact with the parts. Careful cleanliness, and the use of nitrate of silver, will get them well; but if there be much neglect, one of these ulcers may become peculiarly obstinate and painful, as in the ordinary irritable ulcer, and require division.

CPSIA,information can be obtained
at www.ICGtesting.com
Printed in the USA
BVHW04*0344200918
527708BV00051B/1668/P

9 780265 960899